W9-CLC-391

CONTENTS

(v) indicates recipes that are vegan or contain a vegan alternative

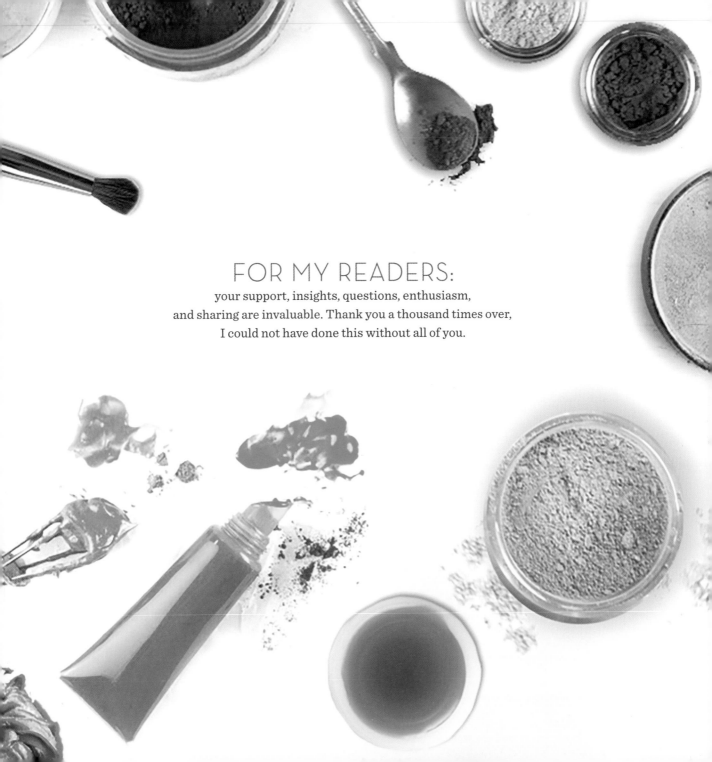

FOR MY READERS:

your support, insights, questions, enthusiasm,
and sharing are invaluable. Thank you a thousand times over,
I could not have done this without all of you.

INTRODUCTION

Safe, natural cosmetics should not be expensive or hard to come by—they're easy to make at home from inexpensive ingredients. With a bit of basic knowledge, some good recipes, and a selection of minerals and plant-based oils, you can ditch the drugstore and the beauty counter and whip up exactly what you need in your own kitchen.

I got my start with homemade natural bath and body products when a close friend wrote her thesis on the migration of chemicals from our body products into our bodies. She shared her findings and I was horrified. There were carcinogenic preservatives in my lotions, irritating synthetic surfactants in my shampoo, and petroleum products in just about everything. Yikes. I considered myself to be a careful person—somebody who read the labels of everything in the grocery store and made almost everything I ate from scratch—and yet I'd never really thought about what I was putting on my body, only in it.

A bottle of argan oil started my love affair with natural ingredients, and from there I branched out to shea butter, beeswax, cocoa butter, jojoba oil, and essential oils. With each new ingredient I tried a new creation—first lip balm, then body butter, lotion, and soap. All were easier than I'd ever imagined, and I loved having total control over my creations. I was hooked, and I want to get you hooked, too.

Getting into making your own cosmetics is a lot like deciding to try out a new cuisine. You love curry, but your Indian buffet habit is getting a bit out of hand, so when a cookbook with beautiful spices and creamy curries adorning the cover grabs your eye, you decide to start making your own. A few of the ingredients sound familiar, but some of them are totally foreign. Your neighborhood grocery store doesn't carry fenugreek or nigella seeds, and their coconut milk seems awfully expensive.

What you need here is the right place to shop and after that you're golden. The same is true with making your own cosmetics. The different butters, oils, and powders sound a bit strange, and your grocery store won't carry a lot of them, but that's okay. You might have a local shop that sells some of the ingredients you'll need, but I've found that local stores are usually substantially more expensive than their online alternatives, and the ingredients often aren't as fresh.

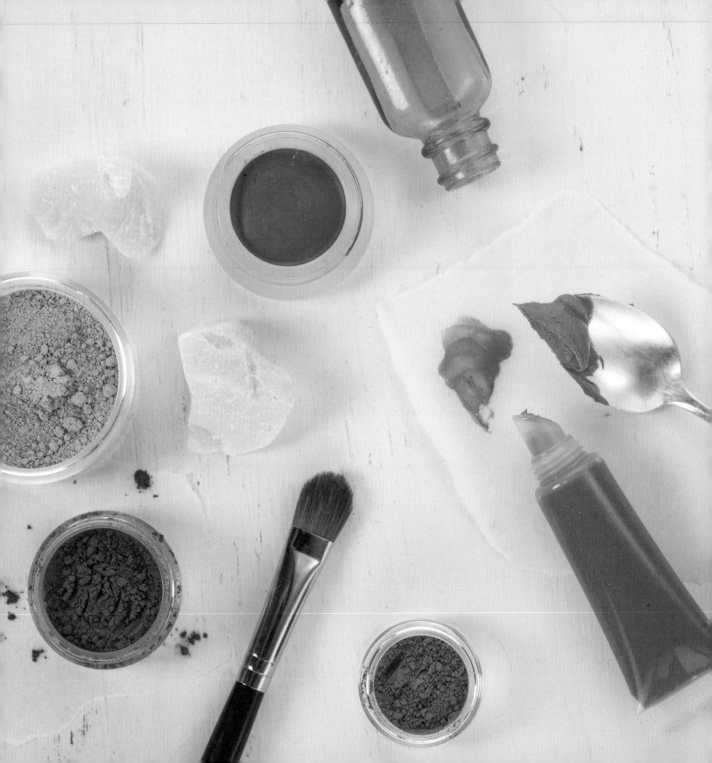

So, you're going to want to shop online when making cosmetics. The selection and variety is fantastic, and the prices are as good as it gets. You'll probably have to pay for shipping, but you'll still save over shopping locally. All that amazing selection can also be really overwhelming, so I've made up some super-helpful starter shopping lists for you (page 35). You'll probably spend about $150, which is roughly the price of a new tube of mascara, a new eye shadow palette, and some mineral makeup that probably doesn't quite match your skin tone. From those ingredients you'll be able to make the equivalent of thousands of dollars of makeup at home!

While you wait for your ingredients to arrive, I recommend a trip to your local thrift or discount store for some equipment. If you already have a well-kitted kitchen, you might not need anything, but if you're interested in doing powdery stuff like mineral makeup, blush, and eye shadow, you'll need to get yourself a dedicated DIY coffee grinder. Flexible silicone spatulas (look for sharp-edged jar spatulas) are also wonderful, and you'll want a selection of pretty jars to put your concoctions into. I've made a list of some kitchen things you'll want to have on hand (page 25).

Once your ingredients arrive at your doorstep, take some time to revel in your self-made Christmas morning. I usually can't resist plopping myself down on the floor with a pair of scissors to chomp through the layers of bubble wrap to my lovely new glass bottles full of exciting new oils and tubs of fluffy, colorful powders. It's awesome.

And now you're ready to dive in head first! Booyah. If you're a comfortable cook, you'll find all of this far easier than you'd have ever imagined. Even if you're not, if you can count, stir, and follow directions, you'll be more than fine. Let's get started!

Tip: Store your ingredients somewhere cool, dry, and dark to get the longest shelf life out of them. I store my ingredients in my basement, but a closet or cupboard that's not right over a heating vent or oven is also a good choice.

WHAT IS MAKEUP?

In the general sense, makeup is a wide array of substances we apply to our bodies to change, alter, and/or improve our appearance.

Broadly, cosmetics fall into three categories. There are creamy, oil-based things like lipsticks, balms, serums, and eyeliner. There are powdery things, like eye shadow and blush, and there are thinner, emulsified things like lotions and toners that contain both oil and water.

Creamy, oil-based things are mostly made from blends of oils, butters, and waxes, with added colorants, scents, and other ingredients to help with slip (how it feels going on) and adhesion (how long it stays on). Store-bought cosmetics will generally use petroleum-derived oils and waxes blended with plant-based ones. We'll be using strictly natural oils, waxes, and butters—ingredients like beeswax, shea butter, cocoa butter, coconut oil, and argan oil.

The pigments and powders that we use to color creamy cosmetics also form the majority of powdered cosmetics. Base ingredients like titanium dioxide, zinc oxide, arrowroot starch, and sericite mica are dressed up with pigments to make a wide variety of different powders for different uses.

Our last category is the emulsion, a blend of oil and water. These concoctions are lighter than their 100 percent oil-based relatives, but also prone to mold as they contain water, so we won't be making too many of them. Homemade lotion is truly a wonderful thing, though, so we'll definitely be making some of that so you can ditch the shop-bought stuff for one that's perfect for you and your skin.

ARE YOU A VISUAL LEARNER?

Check out the Humblebee & Me YouTube channel to see the techniques used in this book in action! www.youtube.com/HumblebeeAndMeDIY

WHAT PROPERTIES DO WE WANT IN MAKEUP?

The three main properties we're concerned with are adhesion, slip, and function.

Adhesion is how long (and how well) the product stays on, and stays put. Anybody who has ever had their eyeliner go full panda on them, or their lipstick turn them into the Joker while they weren't looking, knows that adhesion is important. Ingredients that bring adhesive properties to our cosmetics include magnesium stearate, titanium dioxide, and kaolin clay.

Slip is how the product feels as you apply it. Silky eye shadows, smooth lipsticks, and creamy balms are all examples of cosmetics that have lovely slip, while chalk would be an example of something that doesn't! Ingredients like magnesium stearate, boron nitride, sericite mica, starch, and jojoba oil help our cosmetics feel lovely, rich, and smooth as they're applied to the skin.

And lastly—and perhaps most important of all—function. If a cosmetic fails at its promised function, it has failed, even if it feels lovely going on or stays put all day. Function is a combination of many things: the right ingredients, the right proportions, and the right procedure. All of that boils down to a good formula, and you're holding a book full of them.

CHAPTER ONE

ESSENTIAL INFORMATION

INGREDIENTS OVERVIEW AND GLOSSARY

Argan oil *(Argania spinosa)*

Shelf life: up to two years if stored somewhere cool and dry

Argan oil is one of the rarest oils in the world, and has been used in Morocco for hair and skin care for centuries. Production is often still carried out by local women who earn a living thanks to growing demand for this awesome oil. Argan oil absorbs into the skin quickly, and just a few drops will leave your skin smooth and hydrated. It's also rich in vitamin E, so it encourages healing, and it has a mild, nutty smell.

Because argan oil is reasonably pricey, I tend to use it by itself more often than not, and sparingly in recipes. It's easily my favorite carrier oil, though, for its amazing ability to heal and soften my skin.

Beeswax *(Cera alba)*

Shelf life: indefinite if stored somewhere cool and dry

Beeswax is the lovely, honey-scented wax that honeybees make. I love the natural, golden variety for most projects, but I've found the refined version (usually available as little white pellets) gives more consistent results in cosmetics, where a small variation in the strength or purity of the wax can noticeably impact performance.

Beeswax is a powerful thickener/hardener in lip balms, body butters, salves, and more. It melts around 145°F (63°C), making it an effective solidifying ingredient, even in higher ambient temperatures (unlike cocoa butter, which, while brittle at room temperature, will begin to soften and melt in temperatures warmer than 85°F [30°C]).

A little beeswax goes a long way when it comes to making something solid, and too much beeswax will give you a final product that feels pretty terrible. It'll be hard and sticky, and will skid across the skin instead of gliding. I've found the lowest ratio you'll generally want to work with is one part beeswax to three parts liquid oils by weight, though there are exceptions when you're adding other ingredients.

Boron nitride

Shelf life: indefinite if stored somewhere cool and dry

Boron nitride is an inorganic compound made

from boron and nitrogen, and this slightly iridescent white powder is a miracle worker in cosmetics, both for adhesion and slip. It makes powdered cosmetics feel rich and luxurious. Eye shadows made with boron nitride are rich and creamy, and don't crawl off into oily creases. It is more expensive than many of the ingredients we'll work with, but we won't need much to make a big difference. As with all fine powders, take care not to inhale boron nitride. I recommend wearing a dust mask when blending, and never lowering the added amounts of oil—they are there to weigh down the final powder so it is not as easily inhaled.

Calcium carbonate

Shelf life: indefinite if stored somewhere cool and dry
Calcium carbonate is a very common compound, found in everything from eggshells to rocks to calcium supplements. We're using it in powder form, where it absorbs oil like you wouldn't believe. We'll use it in eye shadows to help prevent creasing and in face masks to pull excess oil out of your skin. Calcium carbonate does have a reasonably high pH of 9.4, so we won't be using it in terribly high concentrations, especially around the eyes.

As with all fine powders, take care not to inhale calcium carbonate. I recommend wearing a dust mask when blending with your coffee grinder, and never lowering the added amounts of oil—they are there to weigh down the final powder so it is not as easily inhaled.

Carmine, powdered
(Dactylopius coccus)
Shelf life: indefinite if stored somewhere cool and dry .
Carmine has been used as a natural red dye for centuries. It's incredibly potent, and I've never found an adequate natural alternative to it. However, it is derived from an insect called the cochineal, so it's not vegan, and there is a bit of an ick factor for some people. It's also quite expensive. Carmine is fantastic in lipsticks, lip glosses, and lip stains, and delivers an amazing red color that's unmatched elsewhere in natural pigments. If you want an artificial (and less expensive) alternative, D&C Red Lake No. 7 is a fantastic color match that can be swapped out 1:1 in most applications (D&C Red Lake No. 7 isn't water-soluble, so it cannot be used in recipes where we're counting on carmine to dissolve in water).

Castor oil *(Ricinus communis)*
Shelf life: up to two years if stored somewhere cool and dry
If you're familiar with castor oil, it's likely as a treatment for constipation. Don't worry—we've got some more dignified uses for it. Castor oil is a thick, viscous oil that is pressed from castor beans. It sits on top of the skin (and lips), protecting them from the elements and adding a glossy shine.

Castor oil also stimulates hair growth, especially when applied directly for an extended period of time. So if you have thin eyebrows, try combing some castor oil through them daily for an inexpensive fix.

Clay

Shelf life: indefinite if stored somewhere cool and dry

There are lots of different clays available for purchase, sourced from all over the world and available in many different colors and varieties. Some are light and smooth, others are heavy and gritty. The powdered clays we'll work with are quite absorbent, making them fantastic for masks (just add water, apply, and let dry) and for cosmetics where you want to combat moisture or excess oil. For cosmetic purposes we'll want the lighter, smoother clays, so we'll mostly be working with white kaolin clay, which is light, inexpensive, and not too drying to the skin.

Bentonite/montmorillonite clay (sodium bentonite) is another clay we'll be working with a bit; it's a weird one! It is highly absorbent compared to most other clays and becomes gel-like when mixed with water, rather than forming a creamy paste. Its molecules also become charged when hydrated, so we want to avoid using metal with bentonite clay so we don't interfere with that charge. Don't worry—the clay won't zap you, and contact with metal won't harm the clay or make it harmful, it just makes it less effective. Bentonite clay also has a relatively high pH (around 9) so we don't want to use it where it might get into our eyes, and people with sensitive skin may find it irritating if it's not blended with something acidic to lower its pH.

As with all fine powders, take care not to inhale clays. I recommend wearing a dust mask when blending, and never lowering the added amounts of oil—they are there to weigh down the final powder so it is not as easily inhaled.

Cocoa butter *(Theobroma cacao)*

Shelf life: at least one year if stored somewhere cool and dry

Cocoa butter is the fat extracted from cocoa beans, and it's a brittle fat, meaning it's hard at room temperature. Think about how hard a nice dark chocolate bar is at room temperature, and that's about the texture of cocoa butter.

It melts at around 93°F (34°C), which is just a few degrees below body temperature. This means cocoa butter is nice and hard sitting on the shelf, but melts beautifully and smoothly on contact with skin. Cocoa butter also absorbs into the skin easily, leaving it smooth and hydrated.

You can buy natural (or raw) cocoa butter, which smells beautifully of chocolate (I've found the strength of the scent can vary a lot by supplier), or you can buy bleached, deodorized cocoa butter, which smells of pretty much nothing. Either will work for your projects. I love the natural variety as I'm always okay with my products having a bit of a chocolaty scent, but which variety you purchase is totally up to you.

Cocoa butter is usually a creamy off-white color, but you can buy dark cocoa butter as well

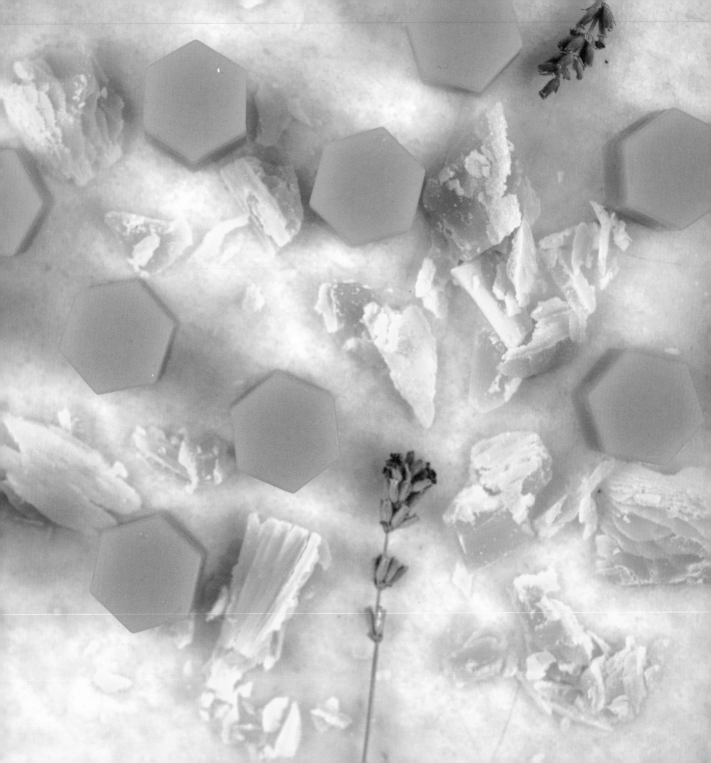

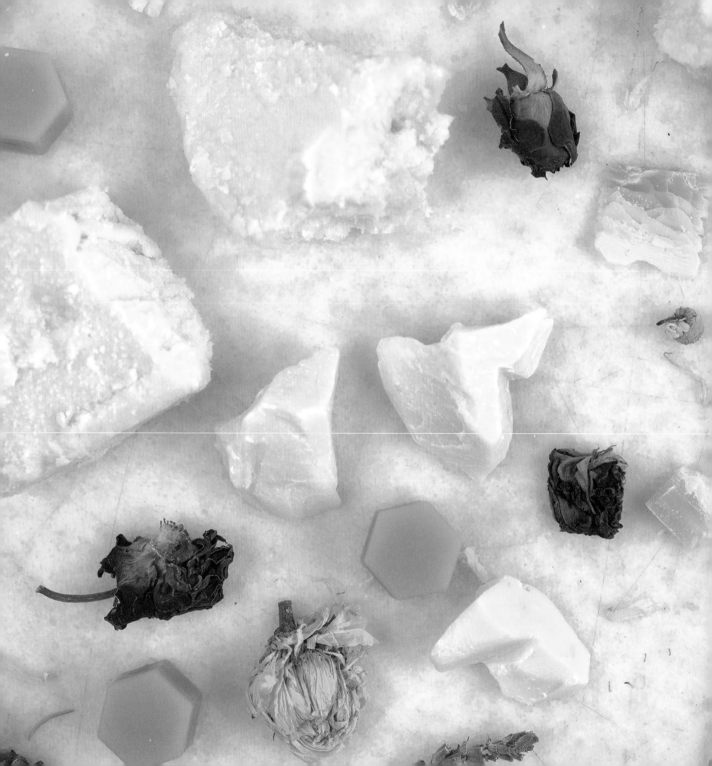

(it's roughly the color of dark chocolate). I've found the dark stuff to be a bit of a novelty as its dark color affects the color of your final product and can stain fabric (just like chocolate), so I'd recommend the lighter variety.

Coconut oil, extra-virgin
(Cocos nucifera)
Shelf life: at least two years if stored somewhere cool and dry
Coconut oil is made from the meat of the coconut, and it's recently become wildly popular as a cooking and beauty oil. It's solid at room temperature in colder climates, but with a melting point of 76°F (24°C), it melts quickly on contact with the skin and is usually liquid in warmer parts of the world. The melted oil is thin and smooth, and absorbs into the skin easily.

You can purchase virgin/extra-virgin coconut oil, which smells wonderfully coconutty, or refined and bleached coconut oil, which has no scent. I highly recommend the extra-virgin version as it imparts a lovely tropical scent into lip balms and body butters.

Coconut oil is also sold with three different melting points; 76°F (24°C), 92°F (33°C), and as a fractionated oil that is liquid at room temperature. You'll want the 76°F (24°C) variety, which is the most common. If you already have some for cooking, it'll be the 76°F (24°C) kind, and you can definitely use it in your DIY projects.

Emulsifying wax
Shelf life: indefinite if stored somewhere cool and dry
Oil and water don't mix without some convincing, and that's what emulsifying wax is for. Emulsifying wax is what we use to make foolproof emulsified lotions (water and oil blended together to create a thick and creamy lotion) as well as cleansing balms, cleansing creams, mascara, and many other things. There are many different brands and formulations of emulsifying waxes, but they all perform the same basic emulsifying function. When used in a recipe at relatively low percentages (this varies by the emulsifying wax) you can easily make lotions that are mostly water (by weight). This makes for a lotion that is lightweight and absorbs into the skin quickly as it's mostly water.

Emulsifying waxes are made from blends of fatty acids like cetearyl alcohol and glyceryl stearate, and emulsifiers like Polysorbate 60. Despite having "wax" in the name, emulsifying waxes perform nothing like beeswax or the c-waxes (carnauba and candelilla), and cannot be substituted for them (or vice versa).

There are two main categories of emulsifying waxes—complete and incomplete. We'll only be using complete emulsifying waxes as incomplete emulsifying waxes require co-emulsifiers to work, and that's far more fussy than it needs to be.

Emulsifying waxes can vary quite a lot in composition and performance. Some thicken faster than others. Some make lotions that feel a bit powdery, and some have longer shelf lives than others. For the projects in this book, I recommend purchasing either Polawax (cetearyl alcohol, PEG-150 Stearate, Polysorbate 60, and Steareth-20), BTMS-50 (behentrimonium methosulfate, cetyl alcohol, and butylene glycol), or Emulsifying Wax NF (cetostearyl alcohol and Polysorbate 60) as we'll be using emulsifying wax to make mascara, and I've found that none of these emulsifying waxes irritated the eyes, while Ritamulse SCG (glyceryl stearate, cetearyl alcohol, and sodium stearoyl lactylate) does.

Note: BTMS-50 and BTMS-25 are not interchangeable, so make sure you get BTMS-50!

Evening primrose oil
(Oenothera biennis)
Shelf life: up to two years if stored somewhere cool and dry
Evening primrose oil is pressed from the seeds of the evening primrose flower, and if you have troublesome skin, it just might be your new best friend. It contains 72 percent linoleic acid and around 10 percent gamma-linoleic acid, two fatty acids that have been shown to be great for acne, eczema, inflammation, dry skin, and dermatitis. It has done amazing things for my skin, and readers have also reported great results. It's a fairly thick oil with a noticeable oily scent, making it well suited to blending with a lighter carrier oil and a

few drops of essential oils to get all of its benefits without leaving your skin feeling heavily oiled.

Grapeseed oil *(Vitis vinifera)*
Shelf life: up to two years if stored somewhere cool and dry
As you might have guessed, grapeseed oil is pressed from the seeds of grapes. It's a wonderfully versatile oil. It doesn't smell like much of anything, it's inexpensive, and it absorbs into the skin quickly with a beautiful satiny finish. I use it in a lot of formulas where fast absorption is key.

Jojoba oil *(Simmondsia chinensis)*
Shelf life: up to two years if stored somewhere cool and dry
Pressed from the seed of the jojoba plant, jojoba oil is a liquid wax that closely resembles our own skin's sebum, making it a wonderful moisturizer. High in vitamin E, it encourages healing and a fantastic complexion. It absorbs into the skin reasonably quickly, leaving a smooth finish. Jojoba oil is also more shelf stable than many other liquid oils, making it a great choice for including in cosmetics.

Jojoba oil is available in a golden and a refined, clear version. Either variety will work for the recipes in this book.

Magnesium myristate
Shelf life: indefinite if stored somewhere cool and dry
This fluffy white powder is made from magnesium and myristic acid (which is a fatty acid).

While it does many wonderful things for your cosmetics, my favorite contribution is adhesion. Magnesium myristate helps your cosmetics stay on your skin for hours without altering the color. It also helps improve slip and finish. You'll find it in lots of eye makeup recipes as it stands up to oily eyelids and hours of blinking very well.

Magnesium stearate

Shelf life: indefinite if stored somewhere cool and dry

Magnesium stearate is a salt of magnesium and the anion of the fatty acid stearic acid (which can be sourced from plants or animals; check with your supplier if the origin matters to you). If you rub a bit between your fingers you will find it to be surprisingly creamy and smooth—not at all like titanium dioxide, which feels pretty dry and chalky. Magnesium stearate is pretty cool. It is oil-soluble and melts at 190°F (88°C). A small amount of it gives face powders and eye shadows a delightfully creamy, smooth feel. It also helps with adhesion, helping eyeliners and lipsticks stay put for hours on end. If you want to press your powders instead of leaving them loose, magnesium stearate is a great binding powder. You'll find it in both powder recipes (like blush and mineral makeup) and oil-based recipes (like lipstick and cream highlighters). The Environmental Working Group's online Skin Deep database rates it at a very safe 1/10.

Micas, colored

Shelf life: indefinite if stored somewhere cool and dry

If you like a bit of sparkle and shimmer in your final products, you'll need some colored micas! They come in a wide variety of colors, but the easiest/cheapest thing to do is to buy white/pearl, and then color it with your oxides.

Micas are mined from naturally occurring deposits before being refined, colored, and sometimes coated with ingredients like dimethicone. You can purchase an entire rainbow of shimmery micas. Some micas are colored with lake dyes and some are colored with oxides and ultramarines—check with your supplier to find out which. As colorful as micas are on their own, they don't pack much of a color punch when you add them to your cosmetics. They're great for added shimmer and tints but for strong, opaque colors you'll need pure pigments.

Running colored micas through your coffee grinder can break apart the pigment from the mica, dulling the effect in your final product. If you're concerned about this (I must admit I am usually not), stir your colored micas into your powdered cosmetics after you've finished grinding everything else together; micas are light enough that they don't need to be ground up to incorporate well.

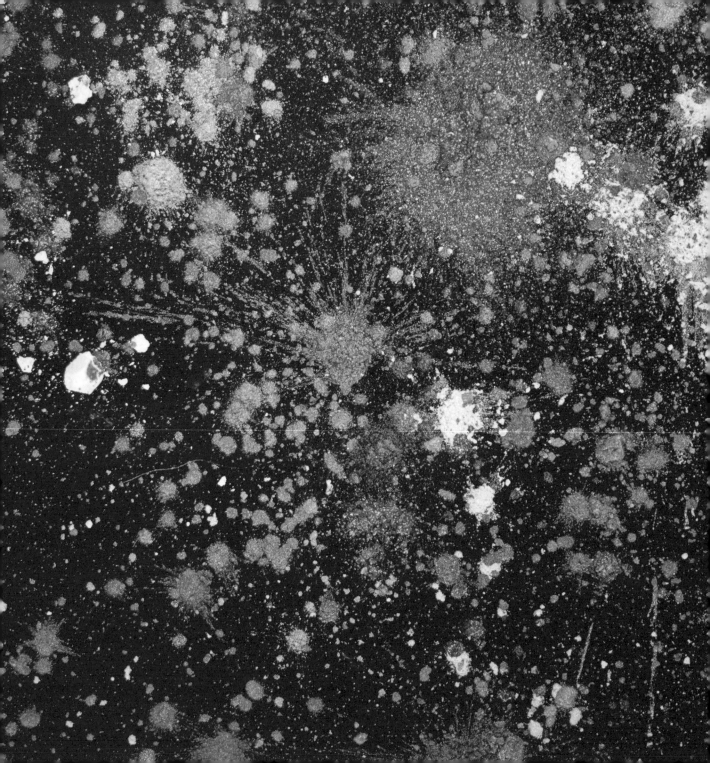

Oxides: iron and chromium

Shelf life: indefinite if stored somewhere cool and dry

You'll definitely want a good assortment of oxides and other pigments—they are what give you color! See page 36 for a guide on which ones to buy depending on the sorts of things you want to make and the colors you like.

Chemically, iron oxides are basically rust—oxidized iron. Don't think your oxides were scraped off an old beater in a junk yard, though—because of contamination concerns with the wild-harvested stuff, cosmetic-grade iron and chromium oxides are synthesized in a lab. It's the same chemical compound that occurs in nature but without the risk of metal poisoning.

The oxides we'll use are powders, and you will find a little goes quite a long way (as such, many of my recipes use measurements well below $1/4$ teaspoon, all the way down to $1/128$ teaspoon—don't worry, though, we'll use special tiny measuring spoons for those). Depending on the color, you will pay $3 to $5 for 1 ounce (28 g), but that generally amounts to approximately $1/4$ cup (60 mL) of powder, and when it is measured out in fractions of a teaspoon, you'll find that will last you ages.

To get the best results from these pigments in powdered cosmetics, you'll need to grind them in a coffee grinder to break them down, evenly incorporate them in the final product and really let the color shine.

Sericite mica

Shelf life: indefinite if stored somewhere cool and dry

Sericite mica isn't quite the same thing as colored micas—it is a fairly unassuming gray powder, and it isn't crazy-glitter-sparkly. It's used as a light diffuser in products, diffusing the light around your skin to slightly blur it, disguising imperfections without smothering them. It also helps with adhesion (how long your cosmetics stay on your skin) and slip. It's a must-have!

As with all fine powders, take care not to inhale sericite mica. I recommend wearing a dust mask when blending, and never lowering the added amounts of oil—they are there to weigh down the final powder so it is not as easily inhaled.

Shea butter *(Butyrospermum parkii)*

Shelf life: up to two years if stored somewhere cool and dry

Shea butter was one of the very first ingredients I started using and I still love it. It's extracted from the shea nut, which is produced by the shea tree that's native to Africa. The smell of the unrefined butter can be a little off-putting to some people (I find it to be vaguely smoky smelling—I don't mind it), but there's always the deodorized variety as an alternative. Shea butter melts at 99°F (37°C), and is soft and a bit sticky at room temperature. It's a great moisturizer, and wonderful in all kinds of projects. If you suffer from dry skin or eczema, try applying it straight from the tub for quick relief.

Silica microspheres (silicon dioxide)

Shelf life: indefinite if stored somewhere cool and dry

Silica is an incredibly common mineral found in everything from bamboo to sand. In microsphere form it's pretty fascinating. If you put this light white powder under your microscope, you'd see a ton of tiny little balls. These teensy spheres lend amazing slip to your products, but they're also incredibly absorbent, making them fantastic for battling excess oil. Similar to sericite mica, silica microspheres also diffuse light, helping give your skin a softly airbrushed look, making silica microspheres a fantastic finishing powder all on their own (some cosmetics companies sell it as such after a massive markup!). Silica microspheres leave your skin both looking and feeling incredibly smooth with a silky, dry finish.

Since silica microspheres can be a bit costly, I haven't included them in too many recipes, though they'd be a great addition to almost anything for added slip and oil absorption. The one place I've found them to be indispensable is in eye primer, where their crazy strong oil-absorbing abilities help keep your eye makeup in place all day. Half a teaspoon of silica microspheres weighs approximately 0.03 ounce (1 g), so if you can purchase 0.35 ounce (10 g) or less, that will be more than enough to make years' worth of eye primer.

If you do want to incorporate silica microspheres into eye shadows, face powders, and other cosmetics, don't run them through your coffee grinder or you'll destroy their sphereness. Instead, lightly mash them together with otherwise finished powdered cosmetics in a sealed plastic bag.

When purchasing silica microspheres, be sure the International Nomenclature of Cosmetic Ingredients (INCI) reads silicon dioxide and doesn't include any mica (or anything else).

Be sure you always wear a dust mask when working with silica microspheres; they're very lightweight and prone to floating around with very little agitation (even opening the bag is enough to send them floating around your kitchen), making them really easy to inhale, which can lead to long-term health problems.

Though the names are similar, silica microspheres/silicon dioxide are very different from silicones like dimethicone, which are synthetic polymers that contain silicon.

Starch

Shelf life: indefinite if stored somewhere cool and dry

Lots of powdered cosmetics include a bit of starch (the same stuff you use in your kitchen to thicken gravy). It's a great, inexpensive, and translucent filler with a silky feel. You can use cornstarch, wheat starch, or arrowroot starch—whatever you happen to have on hand or prefer. I usually choose arrowroot starch.

Sweet almond oil

(Prunus amygdalus dulcis)

Shelf life: up to two years if stored somewhere cool and dry

Pressed from almonds, sweet almond oil is a wonderfully versatile carrier oil. It absorbs into the skin at an average speed and has little scent or color. It's great for irritated skin, and I love it in lip balms. Those with tree nut allergies should obviously avoid sweet almond oil; safflower oil is a good alternative.

Titanium dioxide, oil-soluble

Shelf life: indefinite if stored somewhere cool and dry

Titanium dioxide is the naturally occurring oxide of titanium. It's a light, fluffy, dry white powder (1.1 pounds [500 g] is approximately 1 quart [1 cubic liter] of the loose powder). It appears in a lot of recipes because it is responsible for brightness and opacity, as well as boosting adhesion. In face powders, blushes, and eye shadows it gives you a bright, opaque base to build other colors on top of.

Titanium dioxide is available in both water- and oil-soluble/dispersible versions. For cosmetics, oil-soluble is the most useful of the two, with better adhesion and water repellency.

As with all fine powders, take care not to inhale titanium dioxide. When blending I recommend wearing a dust mask, and never reduce the added amounts of oil—they are there to weigh down the final powder so it is not as easily inhaled.

Ultramarines

Shelf life: indefinite if stored somewhere cool and dry

Functionally, ultramarines act like iron oxides; they're just available in brighter colors. While iron oxides are earthy shades of red and brown, ultramarines are bright lavender (which is usually sold as "pink"), violet, and blue. The original ultramarine (the name comes from the Latin *ultramarinus*, which means "beyond the sea") was an incredibly valuable bright blue pigment made from ground lapis lazuli mined in Afghanistan. A synthetic version was developed in the early 1800s, and now ultramarines are made in labs from a selection of clay, sulfur, sodium sulfate, sodium carbonate, charcoal, siliceous matter, and carbonaceous matter, depending on the color being produced.

Ultramarines are approved for use on the face and eyes in both the United States and the European Union, but they are not approved for use on the lips in the U.S. (though they are in the E.U.). Given the European Union's approval, I have included ultramarine blue in a few lip colors, but if you are uncomfortable using it, FD&C Blue No. 1 Aluminum Lake is a good synthetic alternative that is approved for use on the lips in both the United States and the European Union.

Depending on the color you will pay $3 to $5 for 1 ounce (28 g), but that amounts to approximately ¼ cup (60 mL) of the powder, and when it is measured out in fractions of a teaspoon you'll find that will last you ages.

Vegetable glycerin

Shelf life: indefinite if stored somewhere cool and dry
Vegetable glycerin is a thick, clear, sticky liquid derived from plants like palm and coconut. It's a strong humectant, meaning it draws moisture from the air toward it, which makes it a fantastic addition to lotions and lip glosses. Even though it's water-soluble, it will self-emulsify in some oil-based formulations when blended at the correct temperature. It also tastes sweet, making it a great addition to lip glosses and stains.

Vitamin E oil (tocopherol)

Shelf life: indefinite if stored somewhere cool and dry
Vitamin E is a powerful antioxidant that also helps skin to heal. We'll be adding a few drops of this oil to most of our oil-based cosmetics to help extend their shelf life by warding off rancidity. Most vitamin E oils you can purchase are tocopherols in a base of soybean oil. Some suppliers offer both a USP and a MT-50 Full Spectrum version, with the latter being significantly more expensive. The USP version is great, so don't buy its pricier counterpart.

Zinc oxide

Shelf life: indefinite if stored somewhere cool and dry
Zinc oxide is a naturally occurring inorganic compound. This dry white powder is quite similar to titanium dioxide and contributes opacity and whiteness to our cosmetics (though not as much as titanium dioxide does). It's also slightly astringent, anti-chafing, and soothing, which is why you'll find it as the active ingredient in diaper creams. Though it does occur naturally, the stuff we'll use is produced synthetically to ensure purity and affordability.

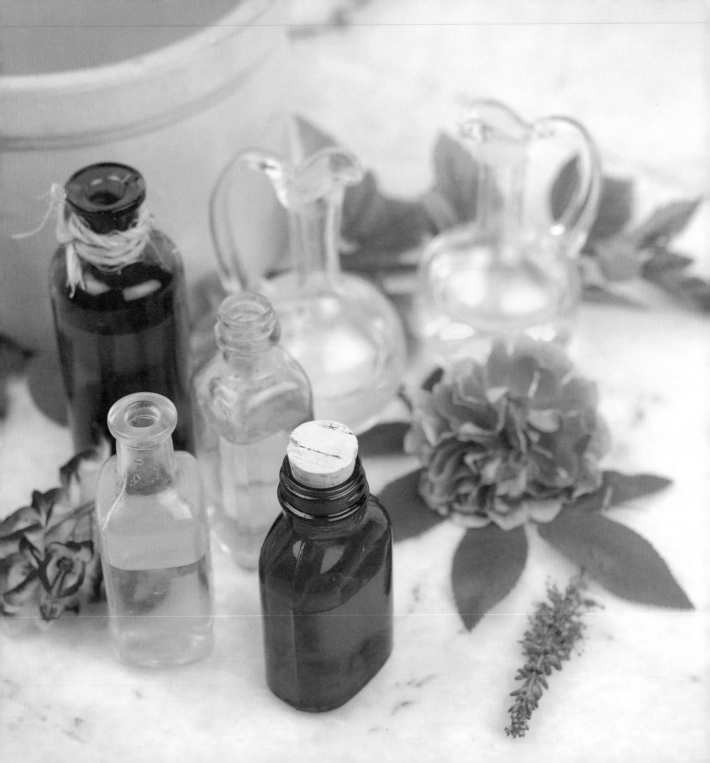

HOW LONG WILL ALL THESE INGREDIENTS LAST, AND HOW CAN I TELL IF THEY'VE SPOILED?

The powders we're working with have indefinite shelf lives, so just keep them cool and dry and they'll be good to use for years.

Oils and butters will eventually oxidize and go rancid, taking on a characteristic smell that's reminiscent of crayons or an old tin of nuts you found at the back of your pantry from a Christmas basket you got back in 2001. To get the longest possible shelf life out of your oils and butters, store them somewhere cool, dark, and dry. If you've got room in your fridge, that's a great place to store more expensive oils, or oils with a shorter shelf life—just let them come to room temperature before using them.

HOW LONG WILL MY FINISHED COSMETICS LAST, AND HOW CAN I TELL IF THEY'VE SPOILED?

With all of our projects we're concerned about two different kinds of spoilage:

If a product contains water, or regularly comes into contact with water, we're concerned about bacterial spoilage—mold, fungus growth, and other disgusting things we don't want anywhere near our skin. We'll ward off this type of spoilage by including broad-spectrum preservatives in these products, but even with those preservatives we can't guarantee never-ending shelf life as our kitchens aren't sterile laboratories. Keep an eye out for changes in color, scent, texture, consistency, and the local mold population; if anything changes, chuck it out and make a new batch.

If a cosmetic is entirely oil-based, or if it's a powder that contains a small amount of oils and no water, we're watching for the oils to oxidize and go rancid. Most oils have a shelf life of around two years, so it's not unreasonable to expect oil-based products to last for at least a year if they are stored in reasonably cool, dry conditions. The inclusion of the antioxidant vitamin E at concentrations around 0.5 percent helps delay oxidization, extending the shelf life of our oil-based concoctions. If you notice any of your lipsticks, eyeliners, or other oil-based products start to smell like crayons or old nuts, that's a good indication that the oils have gone rancid; throw it away and make a fresh batch.

MATERIALS AND EQUIPMENT OVERVIEW

A small saucepan or two

(approximately 1 quart [1 liter] in volume)
You'll use these frequently to melt oils, make lotions, and create a makeshift double boiler with heat-resistant glass measuring cups. Saucepans are easily used for both DIY projects and cooking—there's no need to buy another if you already have one.

A wide, shallow pan

Something like a frying pan or a sauté pan is perfect; you just need to be able to put about 1 inch (2.5 cm) of water into the pan to create a hot water bath to keep little bowls of lipsticks and eyeliners melted while you blend in pigments, and a wide, shallow pan will give you much more room to work than a saucepan. Feel free to use one you've already got in your kitchen, there's no reason to get another.

A 1 cup (250 mL) heat-resistant glass measuring cup

I started with one and found it so useful for melting oils and blending up concoctions that I now permanently hunt for them at garage sales and thrift shops. These cups are infinitely useful for both cooking and DIY projects. All of mine are Pyrex brand.

Some small glass or metal bowls

I've found little custard cups, ramekins, and small glass prep bowls to be wonderfully useful for blending colors, weighing out ingredients, and mixing up small batches of this and that. Look for ones that hold $1/2$ cup (125 mL) or less; you can easily buy sets of them online for around $6. You'll probably see small silicone dishes/cups for sale, but I don't recommend them; because if silicone doesn't heat up, you'll find your cosmetics melt slowly and solidify quickly, making it difficult to blend in pigments.

Flexible silicone spatulas

You can't go wrong with a few of these for blending pigments, stirring ingredients, and scraping the last bits of lipstick out of your pots and pans (added bonus—easier cleanup!). My favorite spatula is a long jar/icing spatula with a thin, flexible edge made by Norpro . . . I have at least twenty!

Metal spoons

The ones from your cutlery set are perfect—brilliant for scooping out coconut oil, clays, and other things that come in tubs.

Miniature wire whisks

You can often buy a set of three or four of these wee whisks for a few dollars, and they're fantastic for making gel eyeliner, mascara, and face masks. In places where a full-size kitchen whisk is far too large, but you still want the blending ability of a whisk, these cute, little ones are perfect.

Standard measuring spoons

You'll want a set of standard baking/cooking measuring spoons—$1/4$ teaspoon (1.25 mL), $1/2$ teaspoon (2.5 mL), 1 teaspoon (5 mL), and 1 tablespoon (15 mL). Feel free to use your normal cooking ones.

Tiny measuring spoons

You might have seen these teensy little measuring spoons at kitchen shops and thought they were an adorable novelty. I've found them to be useful for precisely measuring out potent pig-

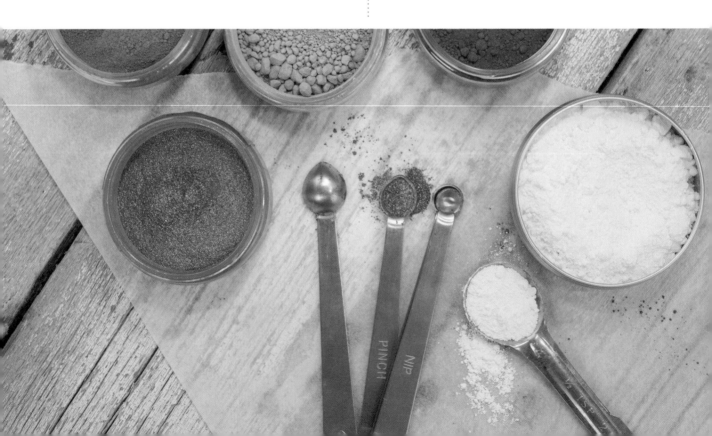

ments. My set contains $1/8$ teaspoon (0.6 mL), $1/16$ teaspoon (0.3 mL), $1/32$ teaspoon (0.15 mL), and $1/64$ teaspoon (0.08 mL). The different sizes are often labeled with cute names like "tad," "dash," "nip," "pinch," and "smidgen," but these obviously aren't regulated sizes, so a "smidgen" in one spoon set can be very different from the "smidgen" in another. If the manufacturer doesn't provide information about what sizes their spoons are in actual amounts, you can do a little test yourself by seeing how many scoops of water (ensure it's a level measure—surface tension can really bung up your measurements) it takes to fill a teaspoon (or half, or even quarter), counting that out, and making note for future use. If you have a scale that can measure down to 0.0003 ounce (0.01 g), you can also use that to check; measure out a level scoop of water and weigh it.

$1/8$ tsp = 0.02 oz = 0.6 g
$1/16$ tsp = 0.01 oz = 0.3 g
$1/32$ tsp = 0.005 oz = 0.15 g
$1/64$ tsp = 0.003 oz = 0.08 g

Some mini measuring spoons aren't based around teaspoon measurements, instead measuring in gram increments like 0.5 g, 0.1 g, and 0.05 g (those weights are for the volume of water the spoon holds). These spoons are a bit short of $1/8$ teaspoon (0.5 g versus 0.6 g), $1/32$ teaspoon (0.10 g versus 0.15 g), and $1/64$ teaspoon (0.05 g versus 0.08 g) respectively, so keep that in mind if you have a set of those instead. I'd recommend not purchasing a set of these measuring spoons and looking for a teaspoon-based set instead.

Measuring cups
You won't need these very often, but your standard set from the kitchen can definitely come in handy.

A digital scale that measures in 0.03 ounce (1 g) increments or smaller, with a maximum weight of at least 1 pound (454 g)
This is an absolute must. Working in weight is so much easier and more reliable than working with volume measurements, especially when you're dealing with solids like beeswax and cocoa butter. Working in weight is the best way to guarantee good results. See page 29 for more tips on buying a scale.

Disposable pipettes/eyedroppers
Many online suppliers will sell these for under $0.05 apiece, and they are wonderfully useful for measuring out drops of liquids.

Little jars and containers
Once your projects are done, you'll need

somewhere to put them. Half cup (125 mL) mason jars are a great place to start, as are empty, old lotion bottles and tins. You can also purchase a wide variety of useful little jars and bottles online (online is definitely the best place to buy lip balm tubes, sifter jars, and jars small enough to use with cosmetics like lipstick and eyeliner, where half a cup is entirely too much). You can also repurpose empty cosmetic jars after a thorough cleaning.

A DIY-specific coffee grinder

Coffee grinders are amazing for making any kind of powdered makeup. They'll blitz together colorants and ingredients better than you ever could with a spoon or a mortar and pestle, giving you a smooth, even blend in no time. A coffee grinder also helps you get the most out of your powdered pigments and mineral ingredients, evenly blending everything and really letting the color shine—the color difference between mineral ingredients that have been ground together versus simply stirred is huge! Use your coffee grinder with a piece of plastic wrap sandwiched between the grinder and the lid to cut back on mess and reduce the volume of the grinder, making for faster, more thorough blends.

You can buy one new (expect to spend $20 to $30) or check your local thrift shop. Look for a reputable brand as cheaper ones will burn out quickly (I've had great experiences with Braun and Krups grinders). You'll also want one with blades rather than burrs, and with a medium-size grinding dish (too small and you won't be able to fit larger batches in it; too large and you'll have to make a lot of every color of eye shadow).

A dust mask

To go along with your coffee grinder and all the fine powders you'll be whirring about in it, a dust mask is a must. Inhaling aerosolized fine powders isn't good for you over the long term, so while you can purchase disposable dust masks, I'd recommend spending $20 to $30 for something bit better. These are your lungs we're protecting, after all!

A funnel

I have a set of three nesting funnels in different sizes, and I use them all the time to get lotions into bottles and lip glosses into tubes.

WORKING IN WEIGHTS: WHY AND HOW

As you flip through this book, you'll notice that a great deal of the recipes feature the ingredients measured by weight (ounces and grams) rather than by volume (fluid ounces and milliliters). This is because weight measurements are overwhelmingly more accurate than volume measurements, especially when you're working with solid, irregularly shaped ingredients. Think about measuring out a cup (250 mL) of gravel by volume—depending on how big the individual rocks are, you'd end up with greatly varying amounts of air mixed in with the rocks, and greatly varying weights, even if the measured volume was technically the same. The precision measuring in weights gives us is extra important when making cosmetics since we're working with really tiny amounts—a jar of lipstick is only about 0.17 ounce (5 g) (and that's still a lot of lipstick!), so a difference of an extra 0.03 ounce (1 g) can make a big difference in the final product.

So, how to weigh? Well, for starters you'll need a scale! Choose a digital one that measures in increments of no more than 0.03 ounce (1 g) (beware of ones that measure in 0.1 ounce [3 g] increments, these are useless for our purposes). If you've already got one that measures in 0.03 ounce (1 g) increments you can definitely use that, but if you're going to buy a new one, I'd really recommend grabbing one that goes down to 0.003 ounce (0.1 g) (or even 0.0003 ounce [0.01g]!). That extra level of precision is fantastic but not necessary. Be sure your scale also has a "tare" or "zero" button as some super-simple ones don't. Scales are readily available online, and you shouldn't have to spend more than $20.

When you get your scale it'll have a couple buttons—usually an on/off (fairly self-explanatory), a "units" button, and a "tare/zero" button. There might be a few others, but these are the three we're concerned with. The units button will generally cycle between grams, kilograms, ounces, and pounds. The weights in this book are provided in both ounces and grams, so choose one of those settings. I'd really encourage you to work in grams, even if you aren't familiar with them. There are 28.3495 grams in 1 ounce, making grams much better suited to the kind of tiny measurements you'll find in this book, and once the scale is working in grams instead of ounces, all you're doing is counting.

The "tare/zero" button will be the button you use the most. It resets the scale to read "0," allowing you to eliminate the weight of your container (and anything in it) while you're weighing out your ingredients. You'll start by placing your container on the scale, and the scale will register the weight of the container. Press "tare/zero" and the scale will read "0" again, allowing you to weigh your ingredients into your container without fussing with any arithmetic to figure out how much of your ingredient you've added.

And that's it—scales 101!

Powdered ingredients are an exception as they measure by volume nicely, and are often so light and used in such small quantities that you'd need a very precise scale to measure them by weight.

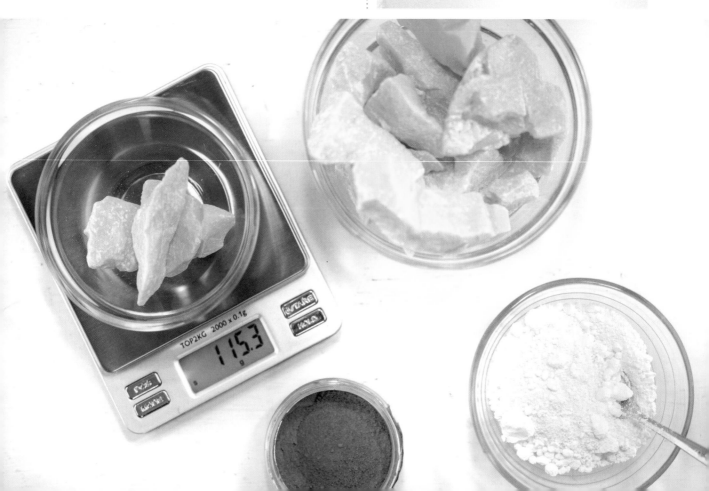

GOOD DIY-ING HABITS

I learned all my good DIY habits by starting off with poor ones, so I hope I can spare you the pain of a lost color blend or mistaken lipstick identity with these tips.

Keep it clean

When we're working at home we can't be sterile, but we can strive to keep things as clean as possible. The cleaner our pots, spatulas, dishes, and containers are, the cleaner our final product will be, and the longer it will last. An easy way to ensure everything is disinfected is by rinsing your tools and containers in a 5 percent bleach solution and letting them dry before making things. Cleanliness is *especially* important when you're making concoctions that involve water, as bacteria loves water.

Measure things

While adding a glug of this and a handful of that is lovely in cooking, those are not recordable, reliable, reproducible measurements for making your own cosmetics. Use proper measurements—weight is best!

Write everything down and take notes

I do mean everything: all your formulas, all your modifications, all weights, measurements, and procedures. Note the date and write down how the recipe performed—and not just when you finished making it, but how is it a week later? A month later? Note-taking is *especially* important when you're blending up colored cosmetics like mineral foundations and eye shadows. Carefully tally up each addition of each pigment so you can recreate your favorite shades effortlessly in the future. You never have to worry about your perfect shade of foundation or favorite shade of eyeliner being discontinued ever again (just don't lose your notes)!

Label everything

No, you won't remember. I've found two-year-old pots and bottles of completely unknown substances at the back of my fridge, and the only thing I remember about them is that I told myself "I'll remember." I didn't, and you likely won't either. I have a set of round brown kraft labels I bought online that I use to label my concoctions, and they work beautifully. Be sure you can tie the name on your final product back to your notes, so you can go back and find out exactly what it is, and consider adding the date you made the concoction to the label as well.

Tip: Your labels will peel right off if there's any oil on your tubes or bottles, so ensure you've wiped your jars down thoroughly with some paper towels before applying them.

Get to know your ingredients

Take the time to handle your ingredients on their own. How do they feel? Hard? Sticky? Slippery? Dry? Coarse? What do they smell like? Knowing what your ingredients are like will help you understand why you're using them (and why you might pair them with other ingredients). It's also helpful if you need to troubleshoot a recipe. Final product too sticky? Perhaps it's the fault of the large quantity of sticky castor oil in the recipe.

Use disposable pipettes

To get the most out of your ingredients and accurately measure recipes that use drops as a measurement, get yourself a dozen or more disposable plastic pipettes. They're usually less than $0.05 a piece, and available in a couple sizes—I like the 0.25 fluid ounce (7.5 mL) ones. Use a different one for each liquid, labeling them using a fine-tipped permanent marker. I like to use rubber bands to secure each pipette to the bottle of its corresponding ingredient to keep everything sorted.

Keep an eye out for spoilage and throw things out when they've passed their prime

We're used to shop-bought cosmetics and body products with seemingly eternal shelf lives, but that's not the case with homemade versions—you've got to keep an eye on them to ensure they're still fresh (see page 24 for more information).

If you observe any changes in color, scent, or consistency, or if you see mold appear in anything you've made, throw it away and make a new batch.

Most of all—be safe

Be sure you're wearing your dust mask whenever you're working with fine powders (*especially* if they're being whirred around in a coffee grinder) as inhaling fine powders can be quite detrimental to your health over the long term. Wear oven mitts when needed, and be very careful with hot oils. Do not leave melting oils and other heating items unattended. Ensure the essential oils you're adding to lip products aren't poisonous (the no-no list includes tea tree, wintergreen, and birch). Work where (and when) small hands and curious paws can't get into things. And above all, use common sense, working slowly and carefully to avoid accidents.

CLEANUP TIPS

Cleaning up after yourself is never fun, but with a few simple tips and techniques you'll find cleaning up DIY messes to be a snap (or at least not truly awful).

First off, preventing a mess is significantly better than cleaning one up. Put old newspapers down over your countertops, especially if your countertops can stain (exposed tile grout, I'm looking at you!). Use smaller dishes rather than larger ones—larger dishes have more surface area that will need to be scrubbed later. Work carefully to avoid spills and splatters, and try to work at a time when you know you'll have your workspace to yourself so no tiny hands or wagging tails foil your efforts at neatness.

No matter how neat you are, you'll always need to clean out the pan/bowl/measuring cup you are melting and mixing in after you move your newfangled concoction into tubes and jars. Kickstart this process by getting as much of your concoction into your final container as possible—I've found thin, flexible silicone spatulas (often sold as jar or icing spatulas) to be brilliant for this. They let you scrape every last bit of lipstick/eyeliner/concealer out of that dish and into your jar, meaning more useable lipstick, and less mess!

Now for the actual dishes part. You'll want to use a straight-up dish detergent here—something powered by surfactants, not natural soap. This is the sort of mess surfactants were made for.

Be careful not to wash large amounts of molten cosmetics down your sink—especially if they contain wax. We don't want them solidifying somewhere in your pipes! That's a big part of why it's best to get your pots down to just streaks of cosmetics, and not clumps.

Powdered cosmetics clean up quite nicely with some dishwashing detergent and a sponge. Oils (particularly anything that's highly pigmented) present the biggest mess. If there's quite a lot of excess left in your dishes, reheat them and use a thin spatula to scrape/pour the re-liquified leftovers into the trash or into a container for use (it's still lipstick, right?). You can also give dishes and spatulas a preliminary wipe-down with paper towels. This is rather wasteful, but it's unbelievably useful when you're making highly pigmented cosmetics like lipsticks and eyeliners, which seem to coat everything with a thin, streaky layer of color.

Up next, boiling water is your friend. Keep a hot kettle by the sink. Just-boiled water will strip oily concoctions off the walls of measuring cups and bowls, though you do need to take care not to burn yourself. I like to combine boiling water with my cleaning powder (see sidebar for recipe) for my biggest messes. Place a spoonful of the powder in the bottom of your dish, add boiling water, and let it sit until the water is cool enough that you can get in there and scrub.

When it comes to cleaning out your DIY-specific coffee grinder, avoid the temptation to use the blender-cleaning trick—don't just add hot water and detergent and give it a whir. Coffee grinders aren't designed to have water in their grinding dish and that water will leak down into the motor (I have destroyed at least one coffee grinder doing this). I find it's best to use a brush to get as much powder as possible out of the grinder. You can also pop a tablespoon of rice in the grinder and blend that up before brushing it out; the powdered rice does a great job of picking up leftover pigments. Use a paper towel (moistened, if needed) to wipe out the grinding dish, and then wash the lid with soap and water in the sink. You'll never get your grinder clean enough to use with food again, but that's okay.

If your coffee grinder stops whirring when you use it and starts shrieking and squealing, chances are it needs a bit of lubrication—blending up all those powders can really dry out the grinder shaft. To get your grinder whirring again, apply a drop of lubricant (I like WD-40) to a cotton bud and massage it around the base of the grinding shaft, between the blades and the grinding dish. Give your grinder a good whir until it sounds healthy again, adding another drop of lubricant if need be. Clean your grinder afterward by blending a few spoonfuls of rice to a powder and dusting that out.

Cleaning Powder Recipe

MAKES ABOUT 3¹/₂ CUPS (840 ML)

1 (2-ounce [60 g]) unscented, plain bar soap, roughly chopped

1¹/₂ cups washing soda

1 cup borax

Combine all three ingredients in a high-powered blender or a food processor outfitted with a chopping blade and blend/process into a powder for about 3 minutes. The amount of time it'll take varies depending on the blender/food processor, but when you're done the bits of soap should be about the size of a grain of couscous. Store in a mason jar and use with boiling water to clean up DIY projects, scrub out tea-stained mugs, and conquer other stubborn messes.

Tip: You can find washing soda at most grocery stores in the same aisle as all the laundry detergent.

STARTER SHOPPING LISTS

REQUIRED INGREDIENTS

The ingredients on this list are all you'll need to get you started making all your own cosmetics and skin-care products. If you are more interested in cosmetics than skin care you can pare the list of oils and butters down to beeswax, candelilla wax, castor oil, emulsifying wax, and jojoba oil.

INGREDIENT	RECOMMENDED QUANTITY	EXPECT TO PAY (USD)
Oils, butters, and waxes		
Argan oil, refined or unrefined	3.3 fluid ounces (100 mL)	$9
Beeswax, refined	8 ounces (227 g)	$6
Candelilla wax	8 ounces (227 g)	$4
Castor oil	16 fluid ounces (473 mL)	$2
Cocoa butter, refined or unrefined	1.1 pounds (500 g)	$9
Coconut oil (76°F)	1 pound (454 g)	$4
Emulsifying wax (Polawax, BTMS-50, or Emulsifying Wax NF)	8 ounces (227 g)	$4
Grapeseed oil	16 fluid ounces (473 mL)	$3
Jojoba oil, white or golden	16 fluid ounces (473 mL)	$15
Shea butter, refined or unrefined	2.2 pounds (1000 g)	$8
Sweet almond oil	16 fluid ounces (473 mL)	$5
Powders		
Boron nitride	1 ounce (28 g)	$7
Calcium carbonate	1 ounce (28 g)	$2

Kaolin clay	8 ounces (227 g)	$4
Magnesium myristate	1 ounce (28 g)	$4
Magnesium stearate	1 ounce (28 g)	$3
Pigments (see buying guide, page XX)	1 ounce (28 g) of each	~$3–$7 each
Sericite mica	4 ounces (113 g)	$4
Silica microspheres	0.2 ounce (6 g)	$2
Starch (corn, wheat, or arrowroot)	8 ounces (227 g)	$3
Titanium dioxide (oil-soluble, non-micronized/high micron)	4 ounces (113 g)	$5
Zinc oxide (non-micronized/high micron)	4 ounces (113 g)	$5
Miscellaneous		
Broad-spectrum preservative (see page 52 for buying guide)	1 ounce (28 g)	$10
Vitamin E oil	0.5 fluid ounce (15 mL)	$4
Vegetable glycerin	16 fluid ounces (473 mL)	$5

PIGMENTS

There are a wide variety of pigments out there, and it can be seriously tempting to purchase the entire rainbow, though you certainly don't have to. For most colors 1 ounce (28 g) (or less) is more than enough. That's about 4 tablespoons of pigment, which is quite a lot!

I'd recommend starting with red, yellow, dark brown, and black. This will give you everything you need to create foundation and all other cosmetics in earthy tones. Consider adding green chromium oxide to this starter set if you like greens in your eye makeup or have a red complexion (as green cancels out red).

If you love a wide variety of lip colors, you should consider getting some blue shade red iron oxide, which is a lovely, cool wine–colored pigment that makes fantastic berry-toned lipsticks. For brighter pinks, reds, purples, and corals, carmine is a must. Carmine is a stunning red-pink color that is integral in many lipstick blends, but it's not vegan and it is pricey (expect to pay ~$40 for 1 ounce [28 g], though prices vary with the market). All the recipes in this book that call for carmine call for brightly colored, powdered carmine (you can also purchase it pre-dispersed in oil, but that won't work in powdered cosmetics). If you love the color, but not the price tag, consider purchasing some D&C Red Lake No. 7. The color is really close to carmine, it's a fraction of the price, and it works in most places we'd use carmine (the exception being lip stain).

For brighter colors, take a look at the ultramarines (available in bright blue, a lavender shade that's sold as pink, and violet) and hydrated green chromium oxide (which is a stunning teal color). These pigments are not approved for use in lip products in the United States, but they are approved for use in lip products in the European Union. As an alternative, FD&C Blue No. 1 Aluminum Lake is a close color match for ultramarine blue that is approved for lip use in the United States.

Be sure to check the ingredients list for your pigments to ensure you're getting pure pigment; in addition to pure pigments, many suppliers sell blended pigments in a wide rainbow of colors that are combinations of several different synthetic dyes, ultramarines, and oxides. You can definitely use these blended pigments if you want to, but none of the recipes in this book were developed using them, so keep that in mind if you're trying to match a color blend you see in here.

If you love shimmer, you'll also want to buy some micas. They're available in an incredible array of colors, but I find I use silver, bronze, and gold most often. Micas start around $4 for 1 ounce (28 g), and go up from there depending on the color.

Note: All the pigments we are using are synthesized. The iron oxides, chromium oxide, and ultramarine blue do exist as naturally occurring pigments, but we use synthesized versions to avoid heavy metal contamination and hefty price tags. Lake pigments are also synthesized, but they do not occur in nature. Lake pigments are available in FD&C and D&C colors, which are approved for use in food, drugs, and cosmetics or drugs and cosmetics respectively. Some are made from natural ingredients, but most are synthesized from petroleum products. Lake dyes are generally available in brighter colors than their more natural alternatives, and they behave like iron oxides do in recipes. They also tend to get better safety ratings than iron oxides do on the Skin Deep database (1/10 versus 2/10). I'd encourage you to do your own research to decide if you want to use lake dyes; the Environmental Working Group's online Skin Deep database is a great place to start.

OPTIONAL INGREDIENTS

These ingredients are optional, as most of them are only used in one or two recipes in the book. Check out the recipes that use them to decide if you want to add them to your shopping list.

INGREDIENT	RECOMMENDED QUANTITY	EXPECT TO PAY (USD)	WHERE IT'S USED
Alkanet root powder	4 ounces (113 g)	$5	Alkanet-Infused Tinted Lip Balm (page 149)
Bentonite clay	1 pound (454 g)	$7	Bentonite Clay Anti-Acne Face Mask (page 69)
Essential oils	See buying guide, below		Optional in most lip makeup and skin-care recipes
Evening primrose oil	4 fluid ounces (118 mL)	$12	Magical Primrose Argan Serum (page 65)
Xanthan gum	2 ounces (60 g)	$6	Gel Eyeliner Base (page 133)

A QUICK GUIDE TO ESSENTIAL OILS

Essential oils are fragrant oils that are extracted from plant matter like citrus peels, flower petals, and spices. They vary greatly in price depending on the plant they're extracted from, with rose essential oil ringing in at over $400 for 0.5 fluid ounce (15 mL), while lavender essential oil costs around $4 for the same amount. Essential oils are generally added to body products for scent, as well as any benefits the essential oil is supposed to have. For example, a lip balm might contain peppermint essential oil for a nice minty tingle, and you might add lavender to a lotion for its scent and supposed calming benefits.

You can make every single recipe in this book without any essential oils, but they are a lovely addition to many projects if you decide you want to purchase a few bottles or happen to have some already. If, for example, you are concerned about acne, you could add some tea tree and lavender essential oil to your serums and toners to add acne-fighting properties to your skin care products. If your concern is anti-aging, having frankincense on hand would allow you to boost the anti-aging properties of everything you make. Talk about customized skin care, eh?

When it comes to purchasing essential oils, there's certainly no shortage of brands and suppliers, often with widely varying costs. I recommend avoiding multi-level marketing companies as their products are hugely marked up and their purity can be dubious. Any company that recommends you consume essential oils should also be avoided as the production of essential oils that are not specifically for food (like food-grade peppermint essential oil) is not regulated by any government body to ensure safety or purity. I purchase my essential oils online from the same places I purchase oils and butters, and I've always been happy with the quality (and price).

There are dozens of different essential oils on the market, but here are a few of my favorites. If you were only going to purchase three essential oils, I'd recommend lavender, peppermint, and tea tree.

Lavender (*Lavandula angustifolia*)
Expect to pay: ~$5 for 0.5 fluid ounce (15 mL)

The classic, all-purpose essential oil, lavender is amazingly versatile. Add it to serums, toners, and lotions to help boost healing and fight bacteria that's been known to cause acne.

Peppermint (*Mentha piperita*)
Expect to pay: ~$5 for 0.5 fluid ounce (15 mL)

The quintessential, tingly, cool mint. Fresh, clean, and cold, peppermint essential oil is wonderful in lip balms, lipsticks, and lip glosses. If you find peppermint too strong, you might prefer the softer spearmint essential oil, *but avoid minty wintergreen essential oil as it is toxic when consumed.* If you love the minty tingle in peppermint, look for varieties with at least 35 percent menthol content—that's what causes the chilly tingle.

Tea tree (*Melaleuca alternifolia*)
Expect to pay: ~$5 for 0.5 fluid ounce (15 mL)

Another famous essential oil, tea tree is a wonderful antibacterial addition to serums and toners. *Keep in mind that tea tree oil is toxic if ingested,* and for that reason it should not be used in lip products.

Frankincense (*Boswellia serrata*)
Expect to pay: ~$10 for 0.17 fluid ounce (5 mL)

Favored by the wise men, frankincense is a great anti-aging essential oil.

Cedarwood
(*Cedrus atlantica* or *Cedrus deodara*)
Expect to pay: ~$5 for 0.5 fluid ounce (15 mL)
If you suffer from eczema, try adding a few drops of cedarwood essential oil to facial serums and body lotions.

Rosemary (*Rosmarinus officinalis*)
Expect to pay: ~$5 for 0.5 fluid ounce (15 mL)
With both antimicrobial and antiseptic properties, rosemary essential oil can help battle acne, dermatitis, and oily skin.

WHY AREN'T THERE ANY CITRUS ESSENTIAL OILS ON THIS LIST?

Citrus essential oils contain photosensitizing compounds that make it shockingly easy for your skin to burn when exposed to the sun. Citrus essential oils are bright, deliciously juicy-smelling, and inexpensive to boot, but it's best to avoid them in your skin-care products unless you can find versions (like bergapten-free bergamot essential oil) that have had their photosensitizing compounds removed.

ARE YOU VEGAN?

The only non-vegan ingredients used in this book are beeswax and carmine. Many of the recipes that feature beeswax also have a vegan alternative, either in the form of another base recipe (lip balm, lip gloss, and lipstick) or in a slightly different format (gel eyeliner instead of creamy eyeliner, or powdered blush instead of cream blush). You can try swapping beeswax for candelilla or carnauba wax at about 80 percent (use 0.28 ounce [8 g] candelilla wax for every 0.35 ounce [10 g] beeswax the recipe calls for), but keep in mind I haven't tested all the recipes with this substitution. Because candelilla and carnauba waxes are harder and glassier than beeswax, cosmetics made with them won't feel quite the same as the beeswax versions.

Carmine is a bright red pigment derived from the cochineal beetle, and in almost all cases, D&C Red Lake No. 7 is a great alternative. It is not a naturally occurring pigment and is synthesized from petroleum products, but it gets great safety ratings on the Environmental Working Group's online Skin Deep database. The only place you cannot use D&C Red Lake No. 7 instead of carmine is in the Snow White Lip Stain (page 161), as D&C Red Lake No. 7 is not water-soluble, while carmine is.

If you don't want to use carmine or D&C Red Lake No. 7, you certainly don't have to—there's still a whole rainbow of colors available from oxides and ultramarines, though you won't find that beautiful bright red note. This means you'll be sacrificing the classic red shades, bright pinks, and bright purples, as red iron oxide is a quite a bit muddier than carmine and D&C Red Lake No. 7.

Both magnesium stearate and calcium carbonate can be derived from vegan and non-vegan sources, so check with your supplier to ensure you're getting a vegan version.

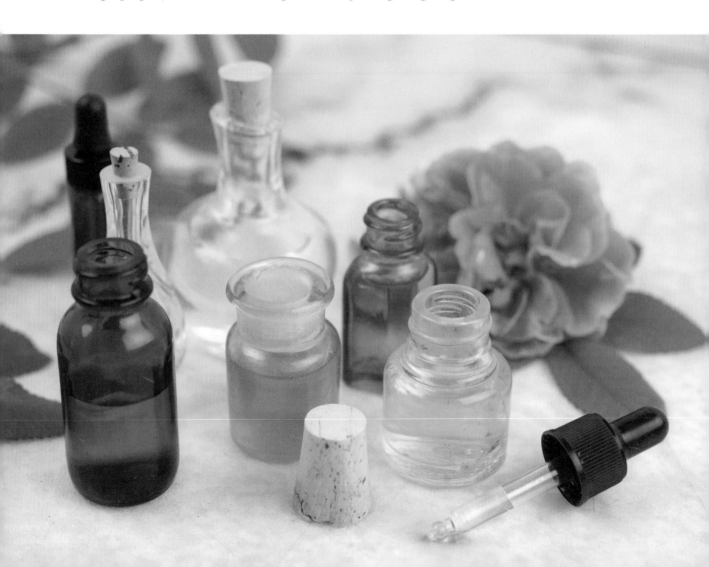

CHAPTER TWO:

STARTER PROJECTS AND CONCEPTS

What kind of cosmetics are there and what do they do? Broadly, cosmetics fall into three categories: oil-based (lipsticks, eyeliners, and cream blushes); emulsion-based (lotions, many foundations, and serums); and powder-based (eye shadows, setting powders, powdered blushes, and more). There's definitely quite a bit of crossover (powdered pigments in oil bases, for instance), but let's look at each category and try some starter projects to get going!

OIL-BASED COSMETICS

Oil-based cosmetics are made from blends of carrier oils, butters, and waxes with added pigments and powders to transform them into cosmetics.

Carrier oils

The term "carrier oil" encompasses hundreds of different oils and butters. In the most basic sense, the word "carrier" serves to distinguish oils that are not "essential" oils—carrier oils are fatty, lipid-based oils. Common carrier oils include olive oil, coconut oil, shea butter, cocoa butter, grapeseed oil, jojoba oil, canola oil, sweet almond oil, walnut oil, and more. Carrier oils vary wildly in terms of texture, color, thickness, nutritional composition, and scent, but generally they are our base oils/butters.

Carrier oils serve a variety of purposes and impact different cosmetic recipes in many different ways. Here's a quick list: bulking/diluting, consistency, speed of absorption, texture, and melting point.

BULKING/DILUTING: The most basic, obvious thing carrier oils do in cosmetics is make up the majority of many of them (along with water in emulsion-based recipes). They are the equivalent of flour or butter in a cookie recipe. If you're wondering "can I just leave it out?," the answer is pretty much always "no." You must replace eliminated carrier oils with something similar, or you will very drastically alter the final product (imagine cookies made without flour!). It will either be too hard, too soft, the pigments will be improperly distributed, and the cosmetic won't function, or, or, or . . . the list goes on and on. Lipstick without oils and butters is just a pile of powdery pigments—not lipstick!

CONSISTENCY: The consistency of an individual carrier oil is based on its state at room temperature, and it brings that consistency to any cosmetic it's included in. Is the oil liquid, soft, or brittle? Each one will contribute differently to a final product (think oil versus butter when baking). One of the most common substitutions people inquire about is using shea butter instead of cocoa butter. This is not a good idea because shea butter is soft and sticky at room temperature, whereas cocoa butter is smooth and brittle, like a bar of dark chocolate. Shea butter will not produce the same smooth, hard final product that cocoa butter will.

If you want to trade one carrier oil or butter for another, your first consideration should be if the replacement ingredient is the same consistency as the original ingredient at room temperature. Your final product will not be exactly the same, but it likely won't fail catastrophically.

This table gives a quick overview of which oils are what, but it's usually pretty easy to tell—especially for liquid oils!

LIQUID OILS	SOFT OILS	BRITTLE OILS
Grapeseed oil	Coconut oil (melts at 75°F [24°C])	Cocoa butter
Olive oil	Shea butter	Kokum butter
Safflower oil	Cupuacu butter	Illipe butter
Argan oil	Mango butter	
Jojoba oil	Babassu oil	
Coconut oil (solidifies at 75°F [24°C])		
Sweet almond oil		
Evening primrose oil		

SPEED OF ABSORPTION: Carrier oils are made up of a wide variety of natural fatty acids, and thanks to that variety, there's a big difference between how quickly different oils absorb into the skin. Some sink in quickly, some slowly, and some very, very slowly. Some oils are "drying" oils, leaving your skin feeling extra soft with no oily residue, and some will leave you so greasy that you won't be able to touch paper for 20 minutes without leaving a trail of greasy fingerprints.

If you want a lotion that you can use on a day-to-day basis without it greasing up everything in arm's reach, you'll want to use an oil that absorbs quickly. If you're making a lip gloss, you'll want an oil that absorbs slowly, so it will sit on your lips and look shiny. If you're making a facial serum and you have oily skin, you'd probably look at using a drying oil instead of a heavy, slow-to-absorb oil.

So, when swapping out oils in a recipe where speed of absorbency is important, ensure the replacement oil is pretty similar to the original in terms of absorption speed. Here's a quick chart of some oil-absorbency speeds.

FAST TO ABSORB	AVERAGE TO ABSORB	SLOW TO ABSORB
Safflower oil	Jojoba oil	Avocado oil
Camellia seed oil	Sunflower oil	Castor oil
Hazelnut oil (also drying)	Argan oil	Shea butter
Grapeseed oil	Sweet almond oil	Evening primrose oil
Rosehip oil (also drying)	Cocoa butter	Oat oil
Apricot kernel oil	Coconut oil	
Canola oil		

TEXTURE AND MELTING POINT: These two characteristics are quite closely tied. Melting point is really only important with oils that are solid at room temperature, as liquid oils generally tend to stay that way when they're out and about (their tipping point into the solid realm is generally far below temperatures you'd want to apply lipstick in—olive oil solidifies around 34°F [1°C], brr!).

One substitution that often sounds like a good idea due to their similar state at room temperature is swapping coconut oil for shea butter, and vice versa. The reason this may not work is a difference in both texture and melting point. In terms of texture, coconut oil is smooth and oily; shea butter is thick and tacky. Coconut oil melts at 75°F (24°C), shea butter at 100°F (38°C) (interestingly enough, cocoa butter melts at 93°F [34°C], even though it is much harder than shea butter at room temperature). Considering body temperature is around 98°F (37°C), this means that coconut oil will liquefy the instant it touches the skin (or in its container on a warm day), while shea butter takes some encouragement. So, in something like lip balm, coconut oil will provide a better glide as it will melt as soon as it touches your lips, while a shea butter lip balm might skid across the lips for the first few seconds (assuming it isn't over 95°F [35°C]).

So, if you are planning on making substitutions in a recipe where the melting point and texture are important, be sure to pay attention to the melting points and textures of your ingredients.

Simple Body Oil

ONE OF THE FIRST PRODUCTS I STARTED USING WHEN I BEGAN DRIFTING TOWARD THE NATURAL/DIY SIDE OF bath and beauty was body oil. Well, technically it was a massage oil that my parents had received as a housewarming gift, but I adopted it.

It was basically just jojoba oil with some essential oils in it, and it was awesome. After argan oil, it was my first experience with applying straight oil to my skin, and I liked it. It was brilliantly hydrating for my dry winter skin, and a small amount went so very far. I carefully rationed that bottle of fragrant oil for months until I finally figured out how to replicate it.

In about 2 minutes this recipe makes a lovely body oil that absorbs quickly into the skin. I've scented it with a few drops of calming lavender essential oil, but you can leave out the essential oil if you don't have it, or use another one that you happen to have on hand (rosemary, chamomile, or cedarwood would all be good choices).

I love using body oil right after a bath, or whenever I need a quick dose of serious, smoothing moisture. It doesn't absorb as quickly as lotion, and its thin consistency makes it best suited for smooth skin (basically not your hands, feet, elbows, or knees).

I decided to blend richer jojoba oil with some lighter grapeseed oil so the finished product would absorb into the skin quickly. If you don't have grapeseed oil, some alternatives include safflower oil, sweet almond oil, and sunflower oil.

The best thing about body oils is that they come together in a flash. Just place all the ingredients in a bottle, shake, and you're done. Nice!

MAKES 1 FLUID OUNCE (30 ML)

4 teaspoons (20 mL) grapeseed oil

2 teaspoons (10 mL) jojoba oil

10 drops vitamin E oil

5 drops lavender essential oil (optional)

Measure all the ingredients into a 1-ounce (30 mL) bottle, using a small funnel to get the oils into the bottle easily. Cap the bottle firmly and shake for 10 seconds to combine. Voilà!

To use, smooth a small amount over dry skin and massage it in. Enjoy your soft, happy skin.

Because this body oil is entirely oil-based, the only spoilage we're worried about is rancidity from the oils oxidizing. Vitamin

E is a potent antioxidant, and will help prevent the oils from oxidizing, so you can expect a shelf life of at least a year if this oil is stored somewhere reasonably cool, dark, and dry. If you notice your body oil has started to smell like crayons or old nuts, that's a sign that the oil has gone rancid, and it's time to throw it away and make a new batch.

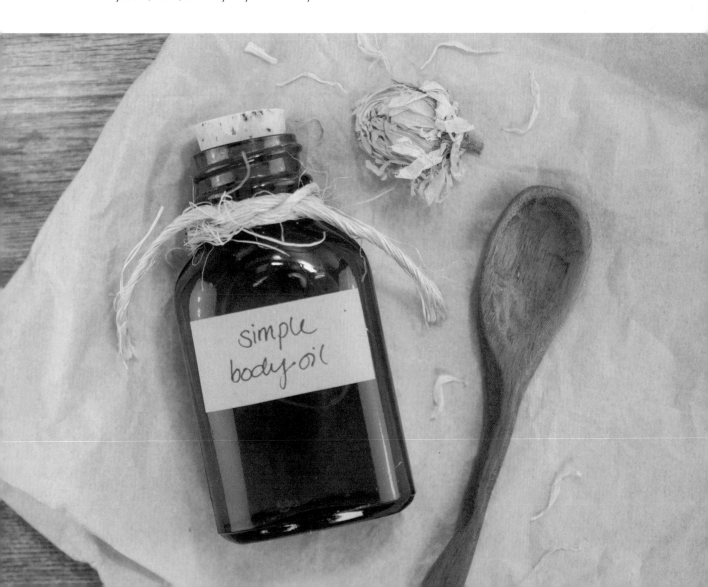

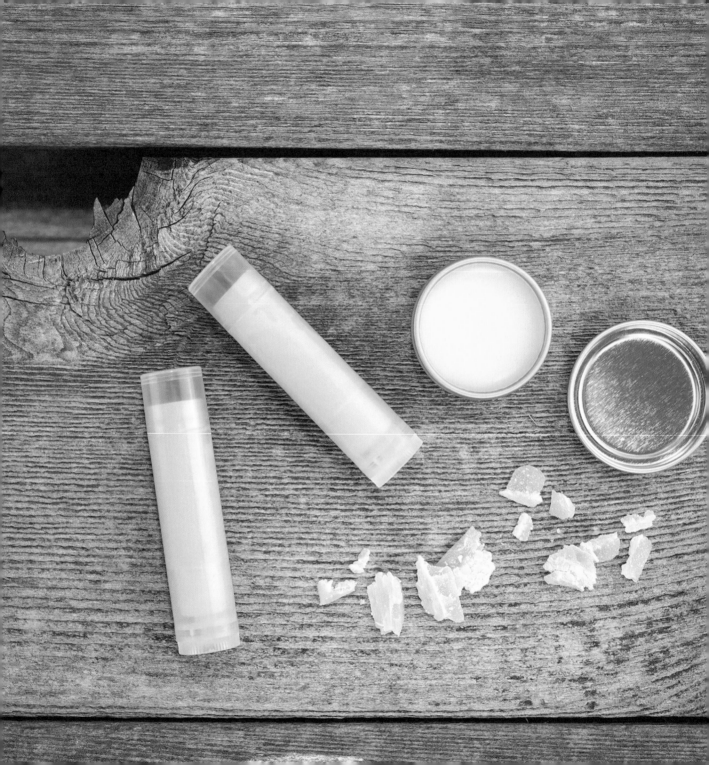

Naked Lip Balm

IF YOU'RE A LIP BALM LOVER, YOU ARE LIKELY FAMILIAR WITH THE PAIN OF HANDING OVER $5 FOR A SOLITARY tube of the stuff. Ouch. If you've ever wondered what on earth makes a few grams of beeswax, oils, and butters worth $5, you are not alone. In the midst of a particularly dry winter in my final year of university I needed lip balm (again), but instead of going to the drugstore, I decided to break my dependence on those little yellow tins and strike out on my own.

It turns out that lip balm is incredibly simple to make, and in no time my dorm room kitchen was pumping out a copious quantity of inexpensive, handmade lip balm. In its simplest form, lip balm is a wax softened with oils and/or butters. The wax is what gives the lip balm staying power—straight oils are too thin to do the job on their own. Beeswax is my favorite wax for lip balms because it's a bit tacky, helping the lip balm stick around. More wax in a formula makes for a longer lasting lip balm, but it also makes for a stickier lip balm that doesn't glide across the lips as well. A good recipe will balance stickiness against staying power, and I'm thrilled to say that this recipe does that beautifully. My Naked Lip Balm glides on and hydrates your lips with a hint of gloss and no irritating tackiness.

I call this Naked Lip Balm because the ingredient list is delightfully bare—in a good way, I promise. Everything you need, and nothing you don't. The lip balm's wonderfully chocolaty, coconutty scent comes from the butters and oils it's made with, so for the best result, use unrefined, fragrant ingredients. No worries if you don't have them (or if you just want an unscented lip balm)—the refined versions of these ingredients will work just as well.

MAKES ELEVEN 0.15 OUNCE
(4.25 G) TUBES OF LIP BALM

0.35 ounce (10 g) beeswax

0.42 ounce (12 g) coconut oil

0.25 ounce (7 g) cocoa butter

0.67 ounce (19 g) sweet almond oil, grapeseed oil, or jojoba oil

6 drops vitamin E oil

Prepare a water bath by bringing about 2 inches (5 cm) of water to a gentle simmer in a small saucepan.

Using your digital scale, weigh the beeswax, coconut oil, cocoa butter, sweet almond oil, and vitamin E oil out into a heat-resistant glass measuring cup (1 cup [250 mL] is a good size for this recipe). Be sure to choose one with a spout for easier pouring later on.

Place the measuring cup in the water bath to melt every

thing together, which should take about 10 minutes. While the oils and butters melt, set out twelve empty 0.15 ounce (4.25 g) lip balm tubes in a row. I find it helpful to have them right up against each other—it means if you spill there's a much higher chance you'll spill into another tube. Be sure you've got enough room around the tubes to pour and maneuver comfortably.

You'll know the beeswax, oils, and butters have melted together when you can no longer see any solid bits in the measuring cup—just a cup of golden liquid. When that's happened, remove the measuring cup from the simmering water and dry it off to prevent accidentally incorporating water into your lip balm, which will speed up spoilage. Stir the oils together with a thin silicone spatula, and then carefully pour the liquid lip balm into the lined-up lip balm tubes. Let everything solidify before capping and labeling—this should take about 10 minutes, you'll know they're solid when the lip balm is opaque and uniform in color.

Because this lip balm is entirely oil-based, it doesn't require any preservatives to ward off bacterial growth, and the vitamin E in the recipe will help delay the oils from going rancid. These lip balms should last at least a year, if not several. Store unopened tubes in the fridge for the longest possible shelf life. If you notice your lip balm has started to smell like crayons or old nuts, that's a sign that the oils and butters in it have gone rancid, and it's time to throw it out and start a fresh tube.

Tip: Are a set of super-dry lips driving you mad? A tacky lip balm can really help as it'll stick around on the lips for ages, locking in moisture. While I find tacky lip balms a bit annoying for daily wear, they're a lifesaver when dry lips are sending me up the wall, and perfect for overnight wear. Whip up a super-simple sticky lip balm by melting equal parts (by weight) beeswax and coconut oil together. Just 0.07 ounce (2 g) of each will fill a single lip balm tube nicely if you just need a wee batch, and you can easily add a couple drops of peppermint essential oil for a bit of minty tingle.

EMULSIONS

You've likely heard that oil and water don't mix—not without a bit of encouragement, at least. To make skin-care products and cosmetics like lotions, body mists, and cold creams, we need to convince oil and water to play nicely together as an emulsion in order to end up with a uniform, creamy final product.

So, what's an emulsion? It's a stable, uniform blend of oil and water—lotion is a great example. To make an emulsion, we'll need an emulsifier—something that brings oil and water together. Emulsifiers are comprised of double-ended molecules; one end grabs water, and the other end grabs oil, binding them together. The emulsifiers we use are also stabilizers, since an unstable emulsion that splits is worse than no emulsion at all.

The biggest advantage of an emulsified product is the ability to include both oil and water, making a product that absorbs much faster than something that is purely oils, butters, and waxes. You can create a lotion that will deliver quick moisture (from the water) and lock it in with the oils, but won't be nearly as greasy as a body butter. Emulsions are also really well suited for hair care, since it takes almost no oil to leave hair looking greasy. With an emulsion you can dilute a small amount of oil in a large amount of water, making it easier to distribute the oil evenly through your hair without immediately needing a shower.

Emulsifiers overview

There are many different kinds of emulsifiers available, but we'll be sticking to complete emulsifying waxes for the projects in this book. You can purchase incomplete emulsifying waxes that require co-emulsifiers to function but those call for quite a bit of extra fiddling, so we'll be sticking to complete emulsifying waxes to keep things simple.

Emulsifying waxes are made from blends of fatty acids like cetearyl alcohol and glyceryl stearate, and emulsifiers like Polysorbate 60—the precise composition depends on the specific emulsifying wax you're using. There are quite a few different emulsifying waxes available, but the four most readily available are:

- Emulsifying Wax NF (cetostearyl alcohol and Polysorbate 60)
- BTMS-50 (behentrimonium methosulfate, cetyl alcohol, and butylene glycol)
- Polawax (cetearyl alcohol, PEG-150 Stearate, Polysorbate 60, and Steareth-20)
- Ritamulse SCG (glyceryl stearate, cetearyl alcohol, and sodium stearoyl lactylate)

Depending on where you live and where you shop, you might find them sold under different names (Ritamulse SCG is sold under several names including Emulsimulse, Natramulse, and Ecomulse), so check the INCI to figure out what you're buying (the list of ingredients that comprise the emulsifying wax, listed above in parenthesis). If you can't get a hold of any of these emulsifying waxes, look for another complete emulsifying wax; check with your supplier if you're not sure. If you'd like to read up on the ingredients that make up your emulsifying wax, the Environmental Working Group's online Skin Deep database is a fantastic resource.

All four of the above emulsifying waxes will work for almost every recipe in the book—the one exception being mascara. I've found Ritamulse SCG to be quite irritating when used near the eyes, so I would recommend purchasing Emulsifying Wax NF, BTMS-50, or Polawax if you want to make your own mascara.

Tip: Despite containing "wax" in the name, emulsifying waxes don't have much in common with beeswax, candelilla wax, and other waxes we use to thicken and harden products like lipstick. As such, they are not interchangeable.

PRESERVATIVES

The biggest disadvantage of emulsified products is the need for the inclusion of a broad-spectrum preservative due to the presence of water. Once water is involved, bacteria are never far behind. We'll need to include a broad-spectrum preservative to prevent the growth of all the different nasties that will try to set up shop in your cosmetics—this is especially true for anything we use around our eyes and mouth.

There are a lot of broad-spectrum preservatives readily available from online soap, cosmetic, and body-product-ingredient suppliers. Here are a few:

- Germall Plus (powder or liquid)
- Optiphen Plus
- Phenonip
- Germaben
- Geogard ECT

The following ingredients are often sold in the "preservatives" section but are not preservatives—just antioxidants. They are usually far less scary/more natural-sounding, but they will not prevent bacterial growth at all. We use antioxidants to help extend the shelf life of 100 percent oil-based products (like body oil and cream blush) by preventing rancidity, but they aren't suitable for preserving anything that contains water.

- Sodium lactate
- Grapefruit seed extract
- Rosemary antioxidant
- Vitamin E oil
- Citric acid

The following preservatives are sometimes listed as broad-spectrum, but are not and require secondary preservatives to work:

- Leucidal Liquid
- NataPres
- NatureCide

Some preservatives are safer than others, and some are easier to use than others. For the projects in this book, I recommend using Liquid Germall Plus. It is an easy to use, water-soluble, true broad-spectrum preservative with a wide effective pH range of 3–8. Used at a 0.5 percent concentration, a little goes a long way to keeping our concoctions mold- and fungus-free.

If you are a more experienced maker and would like to use a different preservative, I encourage you to do extensive research before choosing one. The Environmental Working Group's online Skin Deep database is a fantastic place to research the safety of different preservatives, and the manufacturer of the preservative will provide information on safe and effective usage. Please consider the effective pH range (many more natural-sounding preservatives, like Geogard ECT, have narrow effective pH ranges, so you will have to adjust the pH of your final product), solubility, and anything that might reduce the efficacy of the preservative. NeoDefend, for instance, cannot be used in anything that contains Vitamin C.

When it comes to calculating how much preservative you'll need to add, the first thing you'll need to do is check the recommended usage rate, which the manufacturer will supply. For Liquid Germall Plus, it is 0.5 percent.

To figure out how much to use, simply weigh your final product (remember not to include the container's weight!) and use simple multiplication to figure out what your usage rate is. If your final product weighs 3.3 ounces (100 g) and your usage rate is 1 percent, you would multiply the weight of your product (3.3 ounces [100 g]) by the recommended usage rate (1), and then divide that number by 100. 3.3 ounces × 1 = 3.3 ounces; 3.3 ounces ÷ 100 = 0.033 ounce preservative (100 g × 1 = 100 g; 100 g ÷ 100 = 1 g preservative). For a usage rate of 2.5 percent, that would be 3.3 ounces × 2.5 = 8.25 ounces; 8.25 ounces ÷ 100 = 0.08 ounce preservative (100 g × 2.5 = 250 g; 250 g ÷ 100 = 2.5 g preservative). Technically this will not give us a formula that contains precisely the usage rate of the preservative as the addition of the preservative will slightly skew the definition of a percent, but if you are working with the higher end of the recommended usage rate, you'll still fall within the acceptable range, and with the small batch sizes we're using (and the even smaller amounts of preservative required), we're expecting some margin of error in any event.

Now that you know how much to use, check the information from the manufacturer to see when you're supposed to add it. This is usually at the very end, after you've mixed everything together and your concoction has cooled to room temperature.

That's it—add the recommended amount of preservative, stir it in, and voilà!

Basic Body Lotion

NOW THAT WE HAVE OUR EMULSIFYING WAX AND OUR BROAD-SPECTRUM PRESERVATIVE, WE ARE READY TO make our first lotion. The method we're using here is best suited for small-scale making; larger-scale production requires the use of a heat-and-hold method and more vigorous blending, but I've never found that necessary for small batch lotions for personal use.

Lotions are made from two parts; an oil phase and a water phase. We'll mix and heat the two parts independently, and then combine them and whisk them together to create an emulsion. As the lotion cools we'll keep whisking, adding any cool-down parts like our preservative and essential oils. And that's it! You'll never need to buy lotion again. Brilliant, no?

Because we're dealing with both oil and water, we want to be extra sure everything we're working with is clean; a quick soak in a 5 percent bleach solution is a good way to ensure your measuring cups, whisks, and spatulas are clean. We also want to stick to fairly small batches; even with a broad-spectrum preservative we can't guarantee a super-long shelf life thanks to our less-than-sterile making environment.

MAKES 3.5 OUNCES (100 G)

OIL PHASE
0.25 ounce (7 g) complete emulsifying wax

0.63 ounce (18 g) grapeseed oil

WATER PHASE
2.58 ounces (72 g) just-boiled water

0.07 ounce (2 g) vegetable glycerin

COOL-DOWN PHASE
10 to 20 drops essential oil of choice (optional)

0.018 ounce (0.5 g) Liquid Germall Plus

Prepare a water bath by bringing about 2 inches (5 cm) of water to a bare simmer in a small saucepan. Using your digital scale, weigh your oil phase out (that's the emulsifying wax and grapeseed oil) into a heat-resistant glass measuring cup (I find 1 cup [250 mL] is great), and place that measuring cup in your water bath to melt everything together. This will happen in 10 to 15 minutes, depending on which emulsifying wax you're using. You'll know everything has melted when you can no longer see any solid bits of emulsifying wax in the oils and the oil mixture is not cloudy.

While the oils are melting, weigh out the just-boiled water and vegetable glycerin into another measuring cup or a small bowl, gently whisking them together to help the glycerin dissolve.

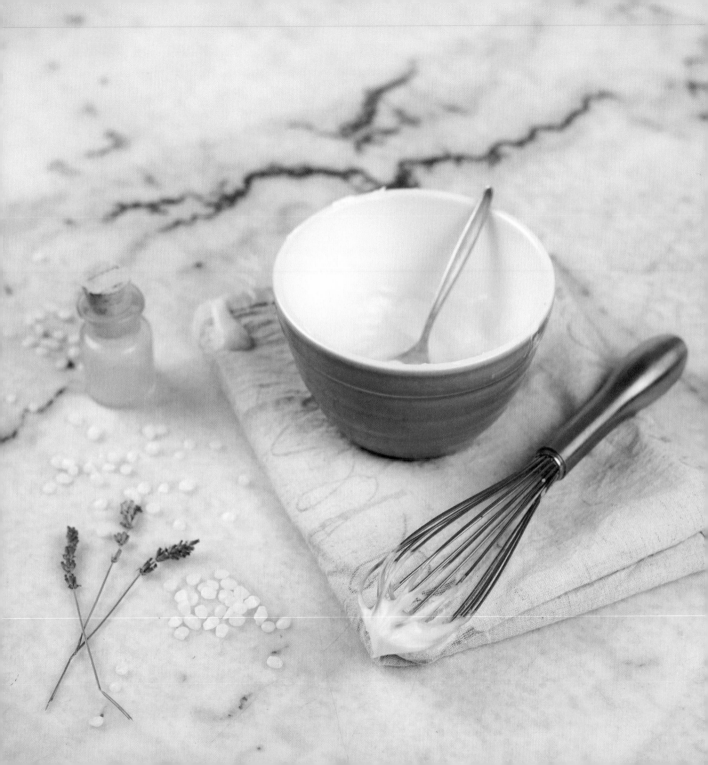

Once the oils have melted, pour the still-hot water and glycerin mixture into the measuring cup of oils, leaving everything in the water bath. You'll notice a blob of white and a sort of curdled appearance—no worries, that's normal. Heat the mixture through for 5 minutes to ensure everything is the same temperature.

After 5 minutes have passed, remove the glass measuring cup from the water bath and whisk the oil/water mixture to combine. You'll see it come together into a lovely white cream within seconds, though depending on the emulsifying wax you used it may not thicken for a day or two. Lotions that are hand-whisked and emulsified with Polawax or Emulsifying Wax NF will have a consistency more like coffee cream than lotion for the first day or two before thickening up, while lotions made from BTMS-50 and Ritamulse SCG will thicken up within the first hour after making. If you have an immersion blender, you can use that instead of a whisk. That will speed the thickening process for Polawax and Emulsifying Wax NF lotions to under an hour.

Continue to whisk your lotion occasionally as it cools. Ritamulse SCG and BTMS-50 require more constant whisking than Polawax or Emulsifying Wax NF for the emulsion not to split, so keep that in mind. Once the outside of the measuring cup is cool to the touch (this will take about 20 minutes), whisk in the preservative and any essential oils you might be using (a blend of lavender and tea tree or rosemary is really nice).

Use a funnel to transfer your lotion to a 4-ounce (118 mL) pump-top bottle or jar and use it in under 2 months. If you start to notice any changes to the lotion in terms of color, consistency, or perhaps even the appearance of a newfound colony of fuzzy mold, chuck it and make a fresh batch.

Tip: The amount of broad-spectrum preservative noted in this recipe equals a 0.5 percent concentration, which is appropriate for Liquid Germall Plus. If you're using something different, check with your supplier to ensure this is an appropriate concentration, as required.

WANT TO PLAY WITH YOUR LOTION?

Switch up the carrier oil you're using! As long as you use 0.63 ounce (18 g) in the end, you can divide it up (try half shea butter, half jojoba oil) and try blends of different oils and butters. Be sure to take notes on all your different concoctions so you can remember what you did when you invent your favorite lotion!

POWDERS

Many cosmetics are powders, or contain powders. The list of powdery ingredients we'll be using is quite long and varied—everything from bright white titanium dioxide to shimmery micas to deeply pigmented oxides. Different powdery ingredients bring everything from opacity to color to moisture management to our cosmetics; let's take a look at the different purposes each powder serves.

INGREDIENT	Opacity	Adhesion	Slip	Moisture Management	Color	Light Diffusion	Bulking
Boron nitride		x	x			x	
Calcium carbonate				x			
Clay		x	x	x			x
Magnesium stearate		x	x				
Micas					x	x	
Pigments	x				x		
Sericite mica		x	x			x	x
Silica microspheres			x	x		x	x
Starch			x	x			x
Titanium dioxide	x	x			x		
Zinc oxide	x			x			

Let's break down the components of the Essential Mineral Makeup (page 84) we'll be making later as an example. For a full-coverage powder, we'll need opacity; this comes in the form of a blend of titanium dioxide and zinc oxide. Unfortunately, these two ingredients are quite chalky on the skin, so we'll add some magnesium stearate (and jojoba oil, though that's not a powder) for slip. A blend of iron oxides makes this bright white, opaque powder skin toned, and sericite mica helps improve the appearance of the skin by gently diffusing light, creating a light "blur" effect. Optional boron nitride adds extra creaminess and slip.

Now let's compare that to blush. With blush we are less concerned about opacity, and more concerned about color. Sericite mica and arrowroot starch make a translucent base for the blush. We'll still include some titanium dioxide for brightness and adhesion (though far less than in the mineral makeup), and we'll add some magnesium stearate for slip and improved adhesion. Then, we'll color the whole lot with some pigments for a pink or red blush.

Working with powders

Measure your powders by lightly scooping them out of the container or bag they're stored in with your measuring spoon, and gently leveling off the top with a knife as you would if you were measuring flour while baking. Don't pack powders into measuring spoons or cups (like you might with brown sugar, for instance) and don't stir or shake the powders up before measuring or you'll throw off the measurements.

You'll want a blade coffee grinder that you use only for DIY projects. Check thrift shops for inexpensive used ones (I've had good experience with grinders from Braun and Krups).

Hold the lid down tightly as you're blending to help prevent powder from leaking out.

Smack the lid of your coffee grinder with the back of a spoon as you work to help knock powders back down into the grinding dish. The powders can crawl up the sides of the grinder and settle down underneath the blades, so you'll need to stir everything around a bit between blending sessions to ensure you're getting a nice, even final product.

Wear a dust mask. It's not good to inhale fine powders, and inhaling large amounts of fine powders can make you sick in the long term. Don't skip the added oils, either; those weigh down the final product so you can safely apply it without it floating out into the air too much.

Don't skip the vitamin E oil, as it extends the shelf life of your powders.

Sandwich a piece of plastic wrap between the grinding dish and the lid by laying it over the grinder and then pressing the lid down onto the grinder as you normally would. This has two huge benefits: it helps seal the grinder so less powder leaks out while you're grinding, and it drastically reduces the volume of your grinder, eliminating the entire lid area. The smaller volume is great for all of our cosmetic projects as it cuts back on the amount of powder you lose to the lid and makes for significantly more thorough and efficient blending. You'll find less untouched powder underneath the grinder blades between blendings, you'll get a far better blend much faster, and you'll make considerably smaller messes.

When adding oils to a powder blend, help them blend in evenly by scattering them over the surface of the powders in the grinding dish rather than clumping them together. I also find it's really helpful to give the grinder a wee shake to shift some dry powder over the oils; this helps keep them from immediately jumping up and sticking to the cling film, giving them a better chance to blend in evenly.

To wash your coffee grinder, brush out as much powder as possible before wiping out the interior with a lightly dampened paper towel. You can also whir a tablespoon of rice in your grinder to pick up any leftover powders. Don't use the blender trick of adding soap and water and blending; coffee grinders aren't designed to blend water and sooner or later that water will seep down into the motor of the coffee grinder and destroy it.

Simple Dusting Powder

THIS SUPER-SIMPLE POWDER IS BASICALLY BABY POWDER, BUT WITHOUT THE TALC (WHICH THE ENVIRONMENT Canada Domestic Substance List classifies as "expected to be toxic or harmful"). I like to use it in the summer to battle sticky legs under skirts, as it's great for preventing chafing of all kinds. We'll blend three simple ingredients together in our coffee grinder and that's it!

MAKES APPROXIMATELY
$^1/_4$ CUP (60 ML)

2 tablespoons starch (corn, arrowroot, or wheat)

2 tablespoons white kaolin clay

4 drops vitamin E oil

Start by putting on your dust mask so you don't inhale any airborne powders. Measure the starch, clay, and vitamin E oil into your DIY-specific coffee grinder. Place a piece of plastic wrap over the grinder, pop the lid on (leaving the plastic wrap between the grinder and the lid), and blend away for about 20 seconds. Rap the lid and sides of the grinder sharply with the back of a spoon to knock down any powder that might have crawled up the sides of the dish, and let the dust settle for at least 3 minutes before removing the lid. Give everything a stir to make sure you're getting an even blend. Chances are some powder will have settled underneath the blades and not incorporated (a stark color difference will usually give this away), or some of the vitamin E oil will have dropped to the bottom of the dish without blending into the powders, so stir all that up and blend again for another 20 seconds. Repeat until you have a uniform, smooth powder.

Transfer your powder to a bottle fitted with a sifter/shaker top; a larger salt shaker (check your local thrift shop) is a great choice!

This powder should last at least a year without spoiling as there's not much in it to spoil as long as it remains dry.

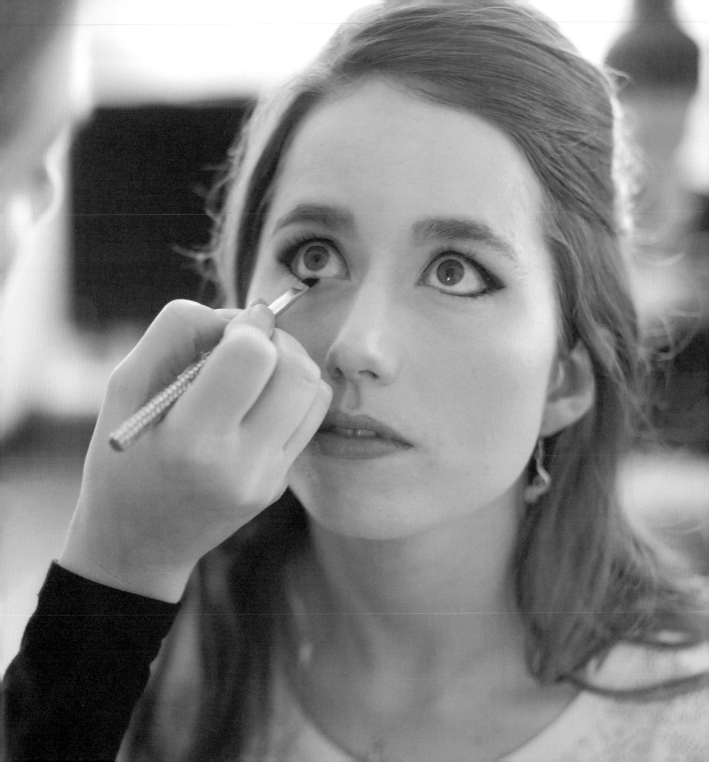

CHAPTER THREE:

SKIN CARE

Beautiful skin starts with healthy skin, and I'm so excited to share my favorite and most popular recipes for healthy, radiant, and clear skin with you. Transitioning to natural skin care can take a bit of adjusting. We'll be trading harsh synthetic foaming cleansers in for natural soaps, clays, and oils; things you've probably been told are too strong for your face, or will make you break out. We'll trade in your oil-free moisturizer for pure argan oil, and your drying alcohol-based toner for tea-spiked witch hazel. Simple clay masks will keep your pores clean and your skin exfoliated, and we'll look at easy ways to customize all these recipes for your skin and your complexion for truly bespoke skin care.

Personally, my skin-care routine isn't fussy in the slightest. It varies with the seasons and by how my skin is behaving (and with whatever recipes I'm currently developing and testing). I'll usually wash my face morning and night, moisturizing with my Magical Primrose Argan Serum afterward. I might wash with a cleansing balm or a clay bar—it all depends on how I'm feeling (we'll chat more about the pros and cons of each method later on). Every week (more or less) I'll do a clay mask for deep-pore cleansing and a bit of exfoliation, and I'm always rewarded with a brighter, smoother complexion. And that's about it, honestly. My skin has improved immensely since ditching shop-bought cleansers and moisturizers, and I love feeling confident about the things I'm putting on my face every single day. I think you will, too.

Essential Argan Serum

ARGAN IS MY ALL-TIME FAVORITE SKIN OIL. IT WAS MY FIRST LOVE IN MY NATURAL SKIN-CARE JOURNEY, and I continue to use it daily. I'll readily admit I was scared of it at first. I'd been told my entire life that putting oil on my skin would make me break out into a pimple-plagued disaster, but my friend Meredith assured me that wasn't the case (she'd used it first), so I gave it a try, and I fell in love. Made from the kernels of Morocco's argan tree *(Argania spinosa)*, it helps boost healing, moisturizes, and prevents breakouts. I'm hooked, and I've got my mom, my best friends, and even old boyfriends on the argan oil train, too. It's good stuff.

You might be thinking the ingredients list for this serum looks a bit short. Aren't serums supposed to have all kinds of fancy ingredients in them? Added vitamins, minerals, and patented mystery compounds to warrant shocking price tags? While all these fancy-pants add-ins are necessary when you start with water and silicone, argan oil naturally contains all kinds of wonderful things. It's rich in vitamin E, an antioxidant that helps skin repair itself. Argan oil has anti-aging properties, and can help prevent acne and balance the skin. It absorbs quickly, leaving your skin soft and hydrated. Argan oil is so potent that you only need a few drops for your entire face. Argan oil is born a serum.

While pure argan oil makes a brilliant serum on its own, you can add a few drops of different essential oils to give it a boost where you might need it. There are essential oils with anti-aging properties, acne-fighting properties, regenerative properties, and more, and you can blend them to add the benefits you'd like to your serum. See my quick essential oil guide on page 38 for an overview of my favorites.

When you're buying argan oil, make sure it's pure—there's a lot of stuff out there pretending to be argan oil that is actually mostly silicone. Read any and all labels, and order from a reputable supplier. Though you can purchase pure argan oil from some cosmetics shops, you'll find it is significantly more affordable if ordered online. I prefer the unrefined version, which has a slight nutty smell. Be sure your argan oil is cosmetic grade as well, as the variety you can purchase at the grocery store is prepared differently, resulting in a much stronger nutty smell.

1 tablespoon (15 mL) argan oil

10 to 20 drops essential oils
of choice (optional)

Measure the argan oil out into a half-ounce (15 mL) glass bottle that has a sealing eyedropper cap, using a funnel to make filling the bottle easier. If you're including any essential oils, add them to the bottle now. Cap the bottle tightly and shake for 10 seconds to combine.

To use, glide a few drops of the serum across your face with your fingers whenever your skin feels a bit dry. I like to use the eyedropper to place a drop on each cheek and my forehead, massaging the oil into my skin with my fingers. I typically use this serum morning and night after washing my face during the drier winter months and less in the summer.

Because this serum is entirely oil-based, it requires no preservatives to ward off bacterial growth, though the argan oil will eventually oxidize and go rancid. Store the serum somewhere reasonably cool and dry to prolong its shelf life—I do not recommend your bathroom. This serum should last at least a year or two, depending on how fresh your argan oil is, but you'll use it all up well before then. If you notice your serum has started to smell like crayons or old nuts, that's a sign it has gone rancid; chuck it and make a new batch.

Magical Primrose Argan Serum

IF YOU SUFFER FROM ACNE OR OTHERWISE TROUBLESOME SKIN, YOU ARE GOING TO LOVE THIS SERUM. With all the concoctions I'm constantly developing and trying, it's rare that something works its way into my daily routine, but this simple blend of argan oil and evening primrose oil has. Evening primrose oil is rich in two special fatty acids: linoleic acid and gamma-linoleic acid. Skin that suffers from acne, dermatitis, eczema, and psoriasis has been found to be deficient in linoleic acid, and studies have shown that adding more of it to your skin-care routine can decrease acne and boost healing. When I first added evening primrose oil to my daily skin-care routine I didn't think much of it until a few weeks later, when I noticed that my skin had been uncharacteristically well behaved. I'd had significantly fewer breakouts, and the ones I did have were smaller than usual and healed far faster than normal. As the months passed, my skin continued to improve with the use of this serum, becoming better than it's ever been. This stuff is incredible; I can't recommend it enough.

Evening primrose oil does have a fairly strong oily scent. Cutting it with argan oil does help reduce that, and adding a few drops of an essential oil of choice will virtually erase the scent.

MAKES 0.5 FLUID OUNCE (15 ML)

1½ teaspoons (7.5 mL) argan oil

1½ teaspoons (7.5 mL) evening primrose oil

10 to 20 drops essential oils (optional)

Measure the oils out into a half ounce (15 mL) glass bottle that has a matching eyedropper lid, using a funnel to make filling the bottle easier. Seal the bottle tightly and shake for 10 seconds to combine.

To use, massage a few drops into the skin with your fingers after cleansing.

Because this serum is entirely oil-based, we aren't worried about mold. This serum should last at least a year before the oils begin to oxidize if stored somewhere relatively cool and dry. If you notice your serum has started to smell like crayons or old nuts, it's time to throw it away and make a new batch—the oils have oxidized and gone rancid.

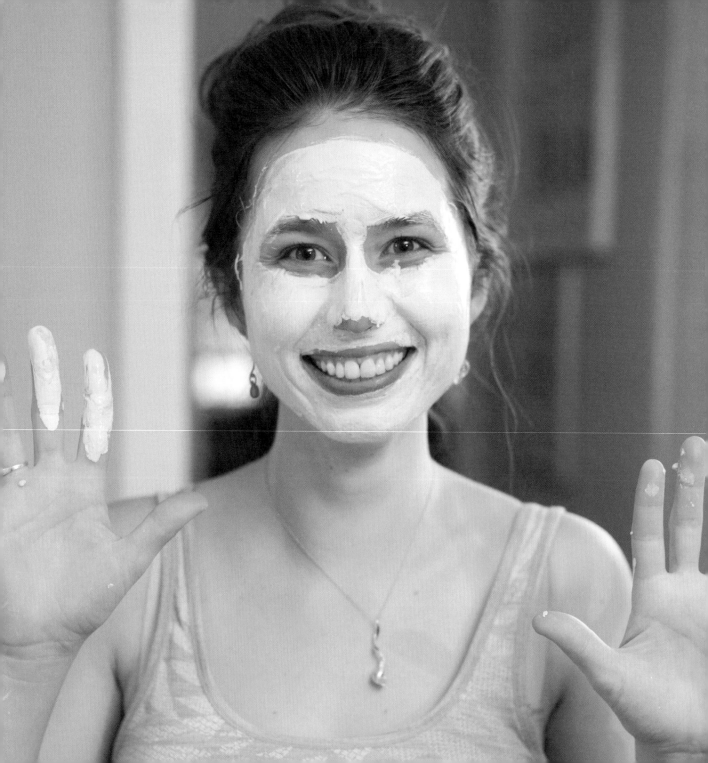

Clay Face Mask

CLAY IS ONE OF MY EARLIEST INGREDIENT LOVES, AND ONE OF MY MOST ENDURING. TURNING CLAY INTO A face mask creates a colorful and amusing pore vacuum that cleans your skin, stimulates circulation, boosts healing, and lightly exfoliates your face when you wash it off. I swear by clay, making a point of doing at least one clay mask a week (or more if my skin is being cantankerous) to keep my complexion clean and bright. While the precise recipe I use each week varies, the overall process and effect is the same.

I'll start by hydrating a clay of choice with some liquid, perhaps adding some essential oils. Once I've got a wee bowl of creamy paste, I'll spread it all over my face and wander around my house looking like an escaped spa client for about 15 minutes before rinsing it off and following up with some Essential Argan Serum (page 63). Easy (and mildly startling for any housemates or delivery people you may encounter with it on)!

MAKES 2 MASKS

- 2 teaspoons (10 mL) warm water or steeped green tea
- ½ teaspoon (2.5 mL) raw honey (optional)
- 6 to 10 teaspoons (10 to 15 g) white kaolin clay
- 10 drops essential oil of choice (optional)
- 5 drops liquid carrier oil of choice (jojoba, argan, or grapeseed are all great choices)

Measure the water or green tea and honey out into a small bowl and whisk them together until the honey has dissolved. Next, slowly sprinkle in the clay, a teaspoon at a time, whisking between additions with a tiny wire whisk or small fork. Adding the clay to the water instead of the other way around guarantees a lovely, smooth mask. The amount of clay you need to add will vary from clay to clay, so simply go slowly and see where you end up—you'll get a feel for it over time. Once you've added enough clay to have a thick, creamy paste, whisk in the essential oils (if you're using any) and the carrier oil. Avoid the temptation to add extra oil, as too much will give you a face mask with the consistency of oily putty! It'll have no interest in staying on your face and will slough off in greasy clods (ick).

Spread the mask over all your face, avoiding your eyes, mouth, and nose. Be sure to cover any problem areas. Let the mask dry for about 15 minutes before washing it off—it should feel tight and look mostly dry. I find starting by soaking a washcloth in warm water and holding it to your face for a few moments to hydrate the mask a bit helps with the washing-off process, as does simply doing a mask before taking a shower. After rinsing off the mask, moisturize your skin with some Essential Argan Serum (page 63) or Magical Primrose Argan Serum (page 65).

CLAY MASKS SHOULD BE USED QUICKLY—IMMEDIATELY, IF POSSIBLE!

If you don't use all of your mask at once, consider reducing the recipe in the future. In the meantime, leftovers can be stored for up to 4 days in the fridge with a piece of plastic wrap pressed right down on the surface. You may find you have to add a wee bit more water when it comes time to use your leftovers, and I recommend letting the mask leftovers come to room temperature before using them as spreading cold clay paste on your face is as unpleasant as you'd guess.

LOOKING FOR WAYS TO MIX UP YOUR FACE MASK?

- Try using a different clay. There's many different types of cosmetic clays aside from kaolin available online, with the most common ones being French green, multani mitti, zeolite, Fuller's earth, bentonite, and rhassoul (or ghassoul). They're all good choices for face masks, though each will require a different amount of liquid to turn them into a creamy face mask. I find red and pink clays can be pretty messy for making masks, so I'd avoid those if you like your towels the color they currently are!

- Use a different liquid, like tea, witch hazel, flat beer, aloe vera juice, fruit juice, milk, or floral hydrosols like rose water. Dilute strongly pigmented liquids (like coffee) or acidic ones (like apple cider vinegar or lemon juice) with water to avoid staining or irritating your skin.

- Swap out 1 teaspoon (5 mL) of water for a teaspoon of fruit or vegetable puree for added vitamins and minerals. Pumpkin, carrot, and apple puree are all great choices.

- For a bit of added exfoliation, add a sprinkle or two of ground spices like cinnamon or cardamom. Avoid anything too irritating, like cayenne pepper.

- Try using a different carrier oil.

- Just remember: if you add food to your face masks, you need to use them up immediately as they'll sprout mold very quickly!

Bentonite Clay Anti-Acne Face Mask

BENTONITE CLAY IS REALLY NEAT. IT'S EXTREMELY ABSORBENT, AND WHEN A TINY AMOUNT IS MIXED WITH water, you'll end up with a gelatinous goo instead of a typical clay + water creamy paste. Bentonite clay's amazing absorbency makes it fantastic for deep-cleaning face masks, and when combined with enzyme-rich raw honey and pH balancing apple cider vinegar, we've got a mask that's brilliant for battling zits and brightening the complexion.

When bentonite clay is hydrated, the molecules become charged, and because of that, we want to avoid contact with metal as it interferes with that charge. Don't worry, you won't get zapped, and contact with metal won't harm the clay or make it harmful, it just makes it less effective.

MAKES 1 MASK

- 1½ teaspoons (7.5 mL) warm water
- ½ teaspoon (2.5 mL) apple cider vinegar
- ¼ teaspoon (1.25 mL) raw honey
- ½ to 1 teaspoon (4 to 5 g) bentonite clay

Stir the water, vinegar, and honey together in a small non-metal dish. I find a single chopstick is a useful non-metal stirring implement for this mask.

Once the honey has dissolved into the water and vinegar, start sprinkling in the clay a tiny bit at a time, whisking as you go. Bentonite is quite prone to clumping, and adding the clay a wee bit at a time and stirring thoroughly between additions helps keep clumps at bay. The addition of vinegar to the liquids also helps prevent clumps from forming. You've added enough clay once you have a thick, frosting-like paste.

Spread the paste on your face, avoiding your eyes, lips, and nostrils, and paying special attention to any zitty problem areas. Let the mask dry for 10 to 15 minutes before washing it off—it should feel a bit tight on your skin. You can leave it longer if you'd like, but 15 minutes is plenty of time to get the benefits of the mask. One of my favorite things about bentonite masks in particular is the dot matrix of pores you'll notice on the mask as it dries—it makes me feel like my pores are getting some serious deep cleaning.

Washing a clay face mask off can be a bit of a messy task. I find soaking a washcloth in warm water and holding it to your face for a few moments to hydrate the mask a bit first helps with the washing-off process, as does simply applying your mask about 15 minutes before getting into the shower. After rinsing off the mask, moisturize your skin with some Essential Argan Serum (page 63) or Magical Primrose Argan Serum (page 65).

Tip: Because bentonite clay is so absorbent in comparison to other clays, it's not a great substitute for other types of clay in a recipe, especially if the recipe contains liquid.

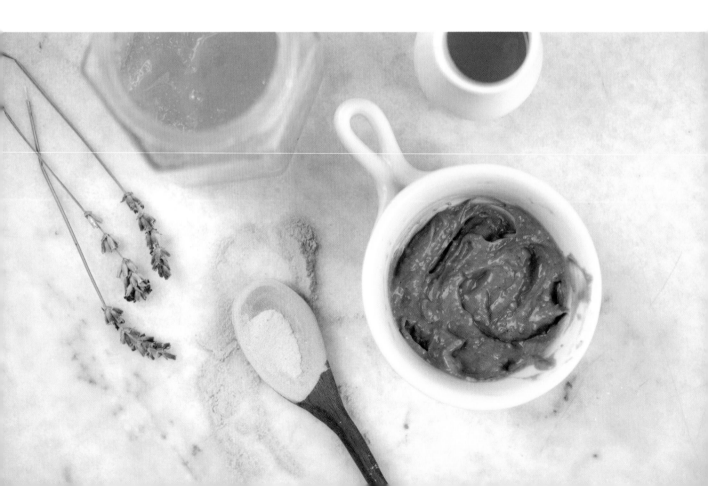

Blackhead Banishing Powder

THIS POWDER IS LIKE A MAGIC TRICK, AND I DO NOT SAY THAT LIGHTLY. JUST YOU WAIT—SOON ENOUGH you'll be recruiting your friends into your bathroom to ambush them with a powdery cotton ball before presenting them with a magnifying mirror to "ooh" and "ahh" over how clean their pores are. Just wait. You'll see.

All of that magic comes from three simple ingredients. It's just white kaolin clay, zinc oxide, and calcium carbonate (which can be bought or made from plain ol' eggshells, which are mostly calcium carbonate). That's it.

White kaolin clay is the base of this brilliant powder. It's a wonderful pore-vacuuming powder on its own (try it in the Clay Face Mask on page 67), and it brings that pore-cleaning goodness to this powder. Up next is zinc oxide, included for its soothing and astringent properties. Last is calcium carbonate, which is a wonderful oil absorber that can be found in everything from toothpaste to eye shadow. And that's it—all you need for some serious pore-scrubbing magic.

Because this all comes together in a coffee grinder to make a fine powder, we need to take some precautions to avoid breathing the powder, which isn't good for our lungs. Please wear a dust mask and refrain from opening the coffee grinder directly after grinding—let it sit for several minutes to give the powder time to settle down before popping the lid off. Once the powder is all done and transferred into a jar, inhalation isn't much of a concern, it's really just the making stage that's a bit of a worry.

MAKES ABOUT ¼ CUP (60 ML)
FLUFFY POWDER

- 1½ teaspoons white kaolin clay
- 1 teaspoon zinc oxide
- 1½ teaspoons powdered calcium carbonate

Combine all three powders in your DIY-specific coffee grinder and blend to a fine, uniform powder (this will take about a minute of grinding), taking precautions not to inhale the powder (see headnote for details).

Once you have a fine powder, transfer it to a wide-mouthed jar. To use, dip a damp cotton ball into the powder and wipe the cotton ball over parts of your face with particularly stubborn blackheads (you'll want to do this part over the sink to avoid getting white powder all over). Let the powder dry on your face until it feels tight (about 5 minutes) before rinsing the powder off and following up with some Essential Argan Serum (page 63).

Tip: Because this powder contains no water and no oils, it doesn't need a preservative or antioxidant. Take care to keep it dry, though—don't go dipping soaking wet cotton balls into it and then sealing it away. Give the powder a chance to dry thoroughly after each dipping.

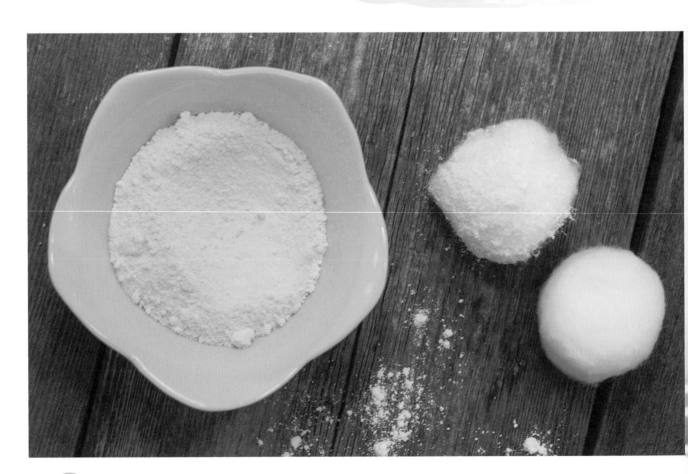

HOW TO MAKE CALCIUM CARBONATE

Feel like going the extra DIY step and turning some discarded eggshells into calcium carbonate? You'll need the shells from about a dozen eggs to get started. You can save these up in the fridge over the course of a week or so, or you could make a big, lovely lemon meringue pie. Rinse the shells and place them on an unlined baking sheet. Bake at 300°F (150°C) for 20 minutes—until they're all dry and a wee bit toasty. At this point you'll be able to pull off and discard any bits of dried-up shell lining (we won't be needing it). Place the shells in your DIY-specific coffee grinder and blitz them into a fine powder. You may need to add the shells a few at a time to make room, but you'll get there eventually, and then you're just be blending away for a while—at least 5 minutes, but up to 10. Take the time to give the powder a very thorough blitzing, as larger bits of eggshell are really scratchy on the skin. Give the powder a test by taking a pinch of it and rubbing it between your fingers and up against your face. If it still feels too coarse, keep grinding.

STORE-BOUGHT VERSUS HOMEMADE CALCIUM CARBONATE

While you can make your own calcium carbonate from eggshells, you can also buy it from the pharmacy as a dietary supplement or from online cosmetic supply shops. Be sure to check the ingredients to make sure the powder is pure calcium carbonate, and hasn't been cut with anything (calcium carbonate pills usually are, so avoid those).

The biggest differences between homemade and store-bought calcium carbonate are purity and mesh (how fine the powder is). The purity of the purchased variety isn't so different from its homemade alternative that you'll notice a difference in performance in this recipe, but you will notice a difference in how they feel against the skin. Shop-bought calcium carbonate will be much finer (think icing sugar versus cornmeal), making for a far smoother final product. Because we'll be using calcium carbonate for oil control in some of the other recipes in this book (including powdered cosmetics that we want to be silky smooth), I'd recommend purchasing some, even if you want to go the eggshell route for the Blackhead Banishing Powder for fun. If you're vegan, be sure to check the source of your calcium carbonate with your supplier, as it may or may not be vegan.

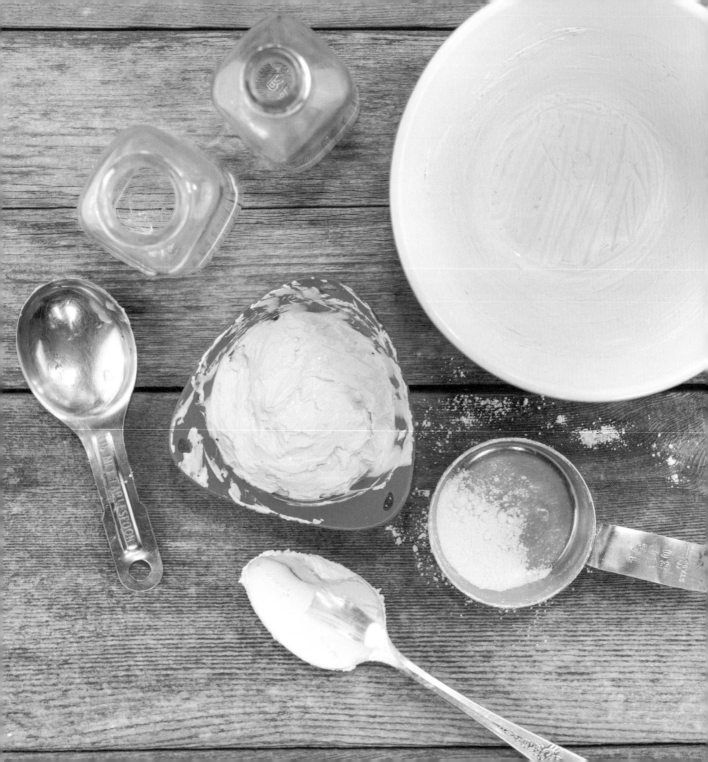

Everyday Clay Bar

A CLAY BAR IS EXACTLY WHAT IT SOUNDS LIKE. CONVERTING CLAY INTO A CONVENIENT BAR FORM MAKES it far easier to apply on a daily basis, and in my life, more convenient = more likely to use. Excellent!

We'll be smooshing dry clay together with just enough witch hazel and high-proof alcohol to form a stiff paste, and then pressing that paste into a mold. Once the bar dries, you'll have a lovely (if slightly lumpy) facial bar that makes adding clay to your daily routine crazy simple.

Something to keep in mind with this bar is the possibility of it sprouting a colony of mold as it dries (which is sad and a bit gross). To prevent this, we want it to dry as quickly as possible (the witch hazel and alcohol help with this). If you live somewhere very humid, I'd recommend setting the wet bar up next to a fan to improve air circulation and speed up the drying process. Also, as tempting as it may be, don't start adding herbs, oils, and other things to the recipe—you're creating a bacteria buffet if you do.

MAKES ONE 1.7-OUNCE
(50 G) CLAY BAR

²/₃ cup white kaolin clay

2 tablespoons + 1 teaspoon (35 mL) witch hazel distillate

2 teaspoons (10 mL) high-proof clear alcohol

Measure the clay out into a medium-size mixing bowl, make a well in the center, and add the witch hazel and alcohol. Stir and mash everything together for 1 to 2 minutes to combine—I like a metal spoon or a stiff silicone spatula for this to avoid getting my hands into the clay paste (once your hands get into it you'll lose a lot of it to your fingers). We're aiming for a stiff, thick paste, so add more clay as needed to get there if the mixture is too wet. You'll be surprised at how far a fairly small amount of liquid goes. Avoid the temptation to add lots of liquid to make a batter that can be poured into your mold as your bar will crack and crumble as it dries.

Once you have a thick, stiff bowl of clay paste, it's time to transfer it to your mold. If you have anything suitable that's made from silicone, like a silicone muffin pan or little egg poaching cups, that's your best option—the drying clay will pull away from the silicone easily, giving you the best end result. If you don't have any silicone options, a $^1/_3$ cup (80 mL) measuring cup works as well (the clay shrinks a lot once it's wet!).

Pack the clay paste into your mold as tightly as you can, and leave it to dry. I recommend coming back to it after a couple of hours and smoothing the top down with the back of a spoon—the clay will have dried out a bit, giving you a more cooperative blob to squish down and level out. If you're using a non-silicone mold, I'd also recommend running a butter knife around the edge of the mold after about 6 to 10 hours to help the bar pull away from the edges evenly as it dries.

Leave the clay bar to dry for a few days in a well-ventilated area, keeping an eye on it. Once it starts to pull away from the edges of the mold you can gently tap it out (this generally takes less than 24 hours) and leave it to dry fully for another few days. You'll know it's dry when the bar is uniform in color, feels noticeably lighter, and is not cool to the touch.

To use, wet your face, and wet the bar under some warm running water. Glide the bar over your face to apply a thin layer of clay to your skin. Let the clay dry on your skin until it feels tight (about 5 minutes) before washing it off—you'll find this clay coating dries much faster than a full mask since there's much less clay.

As long as you allow your bar to dry fully between uses, it shouldn't need any pre-servatives and should last indefinitely. How-ever, if you live somewhere quite humid, where the bar is unlikely to dry quickly between uses, you should consider adding a broad-spectrum preservative as the bar can and will grow mold. Needless to say, if you see any mold, throw it out and make another—this time including a broad-spectrum preservative.

Creamy Clay Cleanser

THIS CREAMY CLEANSER IS BRILLIANT FOR EVERYDAY USE. IT'LL EASILY TAKE A FULL FACE OF MAKEUP OFF without harsh surfactants or eye-stinging soaps, and I find it's gentle enough that I don't need a moisturizer afterward. Made with just four ingredients, it comes together in a flash.

The base of this cleanser is grapeseed oil, a lightweight oil that is pressed from the seeds of grapes. It's high in linoleic acid, meaning it's good for dry or acne-prone skin, and since it's nice and light, you won't feel like you've doused yourself in salad dressing. If you don't have grapeseed oil, sweet almond oil or safflower oil would both be great alternatives. Up next is some emulsifying wax—whichever one you have on hand is fine, as long as it's a complete emulsifying wax. The emulsifying wax is what powers this cleanser. The molecules of emulsifiers have an end that loves water, and an end that loves oil, meaning one end will pick up the oils and bacteria on your face, and the other end will latch on to the water you're washing with and carry it all down the drain. Cool, eh? From there we'll add a bit of white kaolin clay for a cleansing boost.

MAKES ABOUT 1.5 FLUID
   OUNCES (50 ML)

1.44 ounces (41 g) grapeseed oil

0.17 ounce (5 g) complete
   emulsifying wax

1 teaspoon white kaolin clay

20 drops vitamin E oil

20 drops essential oils (optional)

Prepare a water bath by filling a small saucepan with approximately 2 inches (5 cm) of water and bringing it to a gentle simmer.

Using your digital scale, weigh the grapeseed oil and emulsifying wax into a heat-resistant glass measuring cup. Measure out the clay and vitamin E oil and add those to the measuring cup as well.

Place the measuring cup in your water bath to melt everything together, stirring to help things along (this will take about 10 minutes). Remove the measuring cup from the water bath when you can't see any more solid bits of emulsifying wax and stir the mixture well to combine everything. If you've got some essential oils that you'd like to include, now would be the time to stir in a few drops (I'd recommend leaving them out if you're planning on using this to remove eye makeup). *Et voilà!* Now you have a gentle, super-simple facial cleanser.

To use, blend a quarter-size amount in your palm with some warm water—it'll become white and creamy. Thoroughly massage the cleanser into your face, rinsing with warm water when you're done.

Because this cleanser is entirely oil-based, it doesn't require any broad-spectrum preservatives to ward off mold and it should last up to a year if kept relatively cool and dry. If it starts to smell like crayons or old nuts, that's a sign that the oils in it have oxidized and gone rancid; throw it away and make a fresh batch.

Tip: I like to store this in a reusable squeezy silicone bottle, but you could also store it in a pump-top bottle. You'll need to shake before use to mix the clay back in, as it likes to settle out, so keep that in mind when choosing a container. Please avoid jars for this one as we don't want to accidentally incorporate any water into the cleanser by dipping wet fingers into it; that will open the door to mold and fungus growth.

Creamy Cleansing Balm

CLEANSING BALM IS EASILY ONE OF MY FAVORITE WAYS TO GENTLY WASH MY FACE, ESPECIALLY IN THE winter, when it's extra dry outside. It's a soft, solid balm made from lovely oils, butters, and waxes, plus emulsifying wax. You've surely heard that "like dissolves like," meaning that the oils and butters in this balm will help dissolve the oils on your skin, taking dirt, bacteria, and makeup along for the ride (down the drain, that is). The emulsifying wax is what makes this a cleansing balm. By emulsifying oil and water, it helps the water you're washing with carry away all the oils from the balm and your skin. I find this leaves my skin brilliantly clean with just a wee bit of creamy lather, but without an overly dry squeaky-clean feeling.

MAKES 1.94 OUNCES (55 G)

0.53 ounce (15 g) emulsifying wax
0.28 ounce (8 g) coconut oil
0.21 ounce (6 g) shea butter
0.28 ounce (8 g) castor oil
0.49 ounce (14 g) jojoba oil
0.14 ounce (4 g) candelilla wax
20 drops vitamin E oil
15 drops essential oils (optional)

Prepare a water bath by filling a small saucepan with approximately 2 inches (5 cm) of water and bringing it to a gentle simmer over medium-low heat.

Using your digital scale, weigh all the ingredients (except the essential oils, if using) into a heat-resistant glass measuring cup. Place the measuring cup in the water bath until everything has melted, about 10 minutes, stirring the mixture with a flexible silicone spatula to ensure everything is thoroughly mixed. You'll know everything has melted when you can no longer see solid bits of any of the butters or waxes.

Remove the measuring cup from the water and dry the outside of it (this is to prevent any water accidentally getting into the balm, which would cause it to spoil significantly faster). Pour the balm into a 2-ounce (60 mL) jar or tin and let it set up for at least 30 minutes before using. You'll know it's ready to use when it is solid and uniform in color.

To use this balm, simply take a pea-size amount in your

palm, add some warm water, and blend the two together. You should end up with a palmful of white, creamy, cleansing goodness. Massage this into your face, paying special attention to problem areas, before rinsing and wiping it away with warm water and a washcloth.

Tip: This balm also makes a great eye makeup remover if you make it without any essential oils; simply moisten a cotton ball, swipe it across the surface of the cleansing balm, and use that to remove your eye makeup!

Because this balm is entirely oil-based, it doesn't need any preservatives, and should last for at least a year before going rancid. Take care not to add any water to it when you're using it (always use a dry finger, or a popsicle stick), as water will create a delicious little breeding ground for bacteria and can lead to mold growth and other gross things happening in your lovely pot of cleansing balm. If you notice your cleansing balm has started to smell like crayons or old nuts, that's a sign that the oils in it have oxidized and gone rancid; throw it away and make a fresh batch.

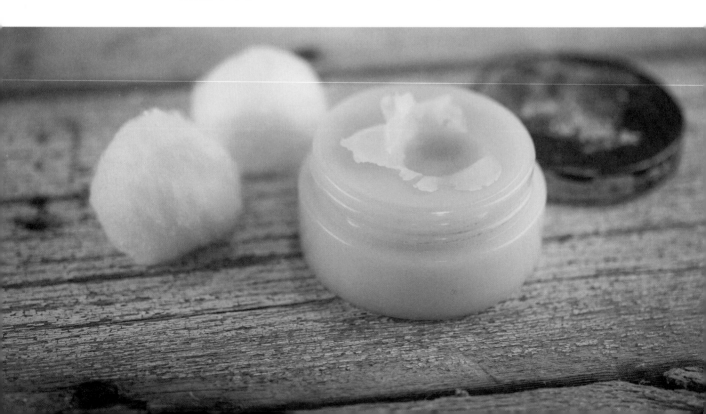

Simple Green Tea Toner

A GOOD TONER IS A LOVELY THING. REFRESHING AND LIGHTLY CLEANSING, IT'LL TIGHTEN PORES AND LEAVE the skin feeling cool and clean.

Toner is, generally speaking, an astringent liquid designed to gently clean the skin and reduce the appearance of pores. We'll use witch hazel distillate as our astringent, paired with some steeped green tea. Feel free to use whatever green tea you might have on hand, even if it's flavored (I love making this toner with a lemongrass-scented green tea for a hint of citrus). Green tea is rich in antioxidants, helping vanquish free radicals and keep skin healthy.

MAKES 2 FLUID OUNCES (60 ML)

1/2 teaspoon green tea leaves

2 fluid ounces (60 mL) water, hot (~176°F [80°C])

1 fluid ounce (30 mL) alcohol-free witch hazel distillate

Broad-spectrum preservative (follow manufacturer's recommendation for usage amount; 1 percent is approximately 0.02 ounce [0.60 g])

Measure the green tea into a tea strainer and place it into a heat-resistant measuring cup. Cover the tea leaves with the hot water and let it steep for 5 minutes.

While the tea steeps, prepare a clean 2-ounce (60 mL) glass or plastic bottle with a sealing cap. Measure the witch hazel into the bottle and set it aside (you'll likely want to use a funnel to make filling easier).

Once the tea has steeped, discard the tea leaves and measure out 1 fluid ounce (30 mL) of the steeped tea. Add the tea and your preservative to the bottle with the witch hazel, cap tightly, and shake again for about 10 seconds to combine.

To use, wet a cotton ball or reusable cotton pad with some of the toner and wipe it over your face, repeating as necessary until the pad comes away clean. That's it!

Because this toner contains water, you'll need to include a broad-spectrum preservative—not an antioxidant. If you notice any changes in color or scent to your toner, it's time to chuck it out and make a fresh batch. If you find you're throwing out more than you're using, consider halving the recipe in the future.

CHAPTER FOUR:

FACE MAKEUP

I am so excited about the recipes in this chapter, and while I'm terrible at choosing favorites, blending my own foundation just might be the best part about making all my own makeup. When I was first discovering makeup, foundation was the most intimidating product out there. Endless bottles of nearly identical beigish liquids and powders lined the drugstore shelves. What color did I need? Was powder or liquid best? It all seemed entirely too fussy, and I usually found I was much too pale for anything on offer, so I'd leave foundation-less, with some eyeliner instead.

When I started making my own makeup, all that changed. I could suddenly create exactly what I needed and wanted. I could finally nail down the right color, choose the level of coverage I wanted, and transform that powder into perfectly matched liquid foundation and concealer. I can make a new batch as my skin tone changes throughout the year, and I'm never worried about my shade being discontinued. I've made foundation for lots of women, and the excitement of nailing down somebody's perfect shade never gets old. Making your own foundation is amazing, and I know you're going to love it.

Once we've got our foundation, we can branch out to blushes, bronzers, highlighters, and color correctors. It's easy to customize the strength and color of everything, so you can always have exactly what works for you. Prepare to feel spoiled!

ESSENTIAL MINERAL MAKEUP

This creamy mineral makeup is where everything starts. You can use it straight, to be sure—it has amazing coverage and leaves your skin looking utterly airbrushed (try it pressed, too: see page 107 for instructions). However, we can also turn this mineral makeup into liquid foundation, high-coverage concealer, and lighter-coverage powders that will all match your skin tone perfectly.

The base of this mineral makeup is a blend of bright white titanium dioxide and zinc oxide, sheer sericite mica, creamy magnesium stearate, and a few drops of jojoba oil. This gives us a bright white canvas to start customizing with yellow, red, and brown iron oxides. The darker your skin, the more oxides you'll need, so the starter color blends for darker skin tones include some additional oil and magnesium stearate to keep the makeup creamy. We'll start slowly, taking careful notes as we add pigment, blending and testing between additions.

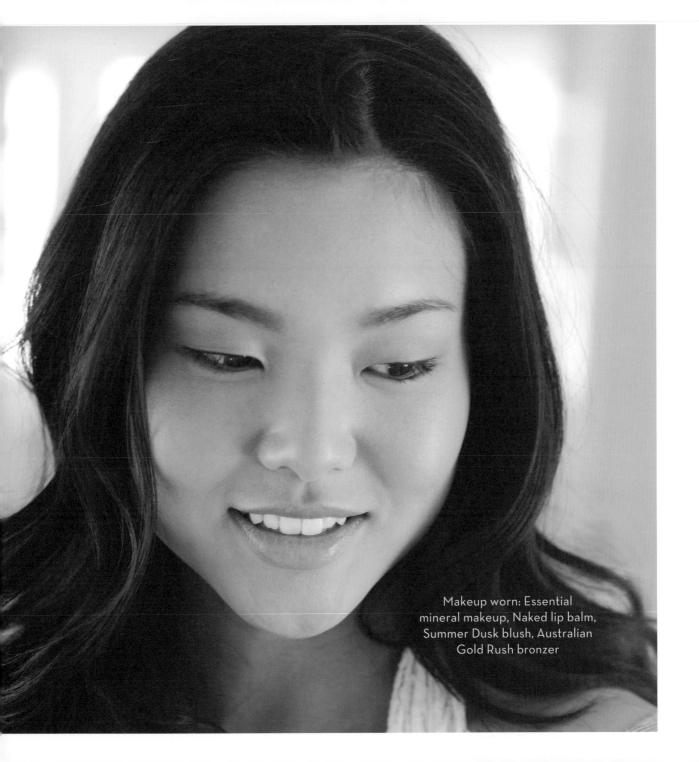

Makeup worn: Essential
mineral makeup, Naked lip balm,
Summer Dusk blush, Australian
Gold Rush bronzer

Essential Mineral Makeup Powder Base

**MAKES APPROXIMATELY
0.42 OUNCE (12 G)**

1 teaspoon titanium dioxide

1 teaspoon zinc oxide

1 teaspoon sericite mica

$^3/_8$ teaspoon magnesium stearate

$^1/_{16}$ teaspoon boron nitride (optional—makes the makeup extra creamy)

20 drops jojoba oil

3 drops vitamin E oil

Pigment (see Essential Mineral Makeup Color Blends section on page 86)

Because we're working with fine powders, begin by putting your dust mask on so you don't inhale the powders.

Measure the powders out into your cosmetics-only coffee grinder, placing a sheet of plastic wrap between the grinder and the lid to reduce leaks and improve your blend. Whir everything together for about 20 seconds. Let the dust settle for a few minutes before removing the lid. Use a spoon to sharply rap the sides and lid of the grinder before removing it to knock down any powder that might have crawled up the side of the grinding dish. Using a small spoon, stir the powders around to see how thoroughly they've blended; some grinders tend to leave a layer of untouched powders underneath the blade. If this is the case with yours, do your best to turn things over with a spoon and blend again for another 20 seconds, repeating as necessary until you have a smooth, uniform powder.

Once your powder base is thoroughly blended, count out the drops of jojoba oil and vitamin E into the grinder, scattering the drops around in the powder rather than clumping them together to help them blend in evenly. I find it's useful to give your grinder a wee shake here to toss a bit of dry powder over the droplets of oil so they blend in rather than immediately sticking to the plastic wrap when you fire up the grinder. Blend again for about 20 seconds, let the dust settle for a few minutes, and then go in with your spoon again and do a bit of stirring. Sometimes the drops of oil plop down to the bottom of the grinder dish and stay there rather than incorporating into the powders, so if that's the case, stir things up, scrape the droplets up off the bottom of the dish as best you can, and give the whole lot another whir.

Now it's time to start adding pigment!

I worked with women of all different skin tones to develop some starter blends, but chances are good you'll need to do some tweaking to end up with your perfect color blend. No worries, it's pretty simple! Choose a color blend that you think might work for you and start with about two-thirds of the pigment called for. Test it on your face and work from there, making adjustments and taking careful notes as you go.

When you're blending in pigments, be sure you're blending for at least 20 seconds at a time. It's important to blend these powders thoroughly to ensure an even color blend. The pigments develop and change quite a lot as they're blended, so short bursts in the grinder won't cut it (nor will just stirring everything together with a spoon).

Once you've created your perfect color blend, transfer your Essential Mineral Makeup to a 1-ounce (28 g) jar fitted with a sifter lid. Because this makeup doesn't contain any water, we're not worried about mold, but the jojoba oil in it can go rancid. The vitamin E in the recipe helps prevent this for at least a year, but if your makeup starts to smell off (like old crayons), it's time to chuck it and make a new batch.

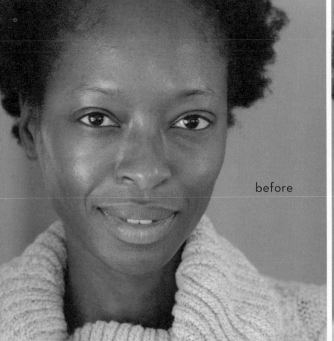

before

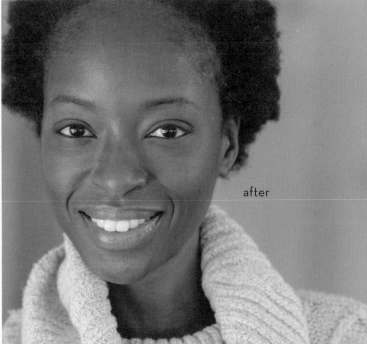

after

ESSENTIAL MINERAL MAKEUP COLOR BLENDS

COURTNEY

Fair with pink undertones.

1 teaspoon titanium dioxide

$1/8$ teaspoon yellow iron oxide

$3/128$ teaspoon red iron oxide

MARIE

Fair with neutral undertones.

1 teaspoon titanium dioxide

$7/32$ teaspoon yellow iron oxide

$3/64$ teaspoon red iron oxide

$2/64$ teaspoon brown iron oxide

JESS

Medium with neutral undertones.

1 teaspoon titanium dioxide

$7/16$ teaspoon yellow iron oxide

$1/64$ teaspoon red iron oxide

$7/64$ teaspoon brown iron oxide

AVNEET

Cool medium.

1 teaspoon titanium dioxide

$7/16$ teaspoon yellow iron oxide

$1/64$ teaspoon red iron oxide

$3/8$ teaspoon brown iron oxide

MONDAY

Dark with yellow undertones.

$1 \, 1/4$ teaspoons yellow iron oxide

$3/32$ teaspoon red iron oxide

$5/16$ teaspoon brown iron oxide

$1/8$ teaspoon magnesium stearate

5 drops jojoba oil

SIMONE

Dark with red undertones.

$11/16$ teaspoon yellow iron oxide

$11/32$ teaspoon red iron oxide

$5/8$ teaspoon brown iron oxide

$1/8$ teaspoon magnesium stearate

5 drops jojoba oil

ADORA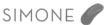

Dark with cool undertones.

1 teaspoon yellow iron oxide

$3/32$ teaspoon red iron oxide

$9/16$ teaspoon brown iron oxide

$1/64$ teaspoon blue ultramarine

$1/8$ teaspoon magnesium stearate

5 drops jojoba oil

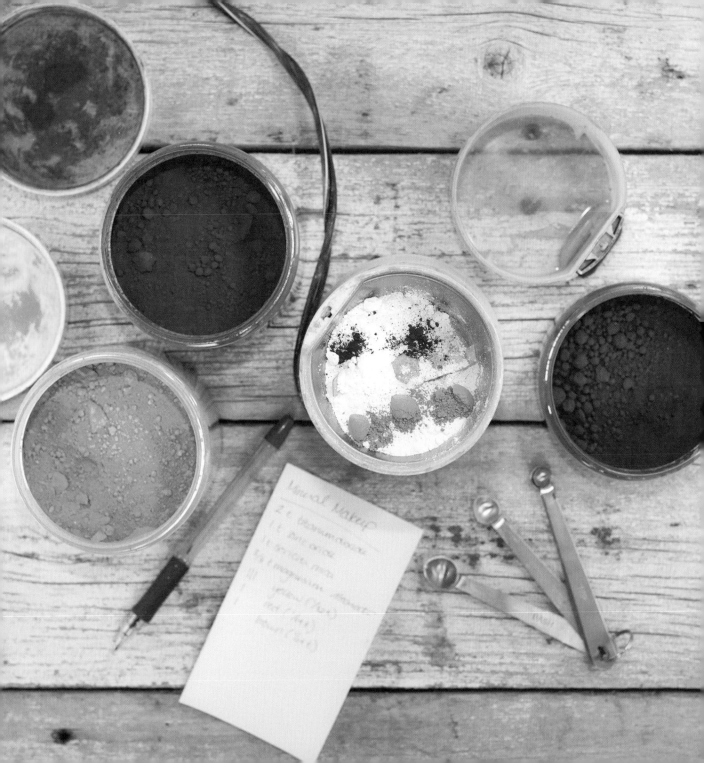

TIPS ON COLOR BLENDING

• Take precise notes, and label all your end products with a name and the date made. My skin tone changes quite a bit over the course of the year, so I'll often have several jars of mineral makeup at any one time that are all slightly different shades of me (this makes for a great customized contour palette!). I find the date made to be wonderfully useful to help me remember how pale each one is (dead of winter = very pale; middle of summer = slightly less pale; etc.).

• Be sure to stir the makeup in the grinder to ensure everything is blending thoroughly; many coffee grinders will leave a layer of untouched powder beneath the blades, so you'll need to get in there with a spoon to mix everything up between blends to make sure you're getting an even and accurate color.

• Not everybody needs brown in their blend, but everyone needs yellow and red. It might not be much red, but I have yet to meet anyone who doesn't need some red to keep them from looking like a zombie.

• Test your makeup on your face (not your arm or hand), using the brush you'll use to apply it (I recommend a kabuki brush). If you're on the paler side, you'll think your makeup looks too dark in the coffee grinder, and if you're darker, you'll think it looks too light. The way it looks in your coffee grinder doesn't matter—try it on your face! Be sure to buff it in as you would if you were properly applying it, too, so you get a real idea of what it'll look like when you wear it.

• If you have got a darker complexion, avoid the temptation to go straight to the dark brown oxide. Remember that the powder base is white—if you only add dark brown to it, you'll get something roughly the color of powdered hot cocoa mix. You'll want to start with mostly yellow, adding brown and red to darken and warm the blend as required.

• Make additions in small increments, keeping careful tally as you go. If you're quite pale, even $1/64$ of a teaspoon of red or brown will go a very long way, so err on the side of caution. You can always add more, but if you overshoot it you'll need to start over.

• You'll need to test your makeup in daylight, so I'd recommend blending it up during the day.

• After a while your entire face will be coated in makeup and you'll need to wash it off to start over with a clean slate. This is a good time to take a break (maybe half an hour) to let your skin relax, especially if you're prone to redness after washing; you don't want to match your makeup to your post-scrub skin tone!

• When you first start testing your batch of makeup, it will always look too light for your skin, but that's not the whole color story. No matter your skin tone, you're likely not using enough yellow.

If you're dark, you're often not using enough pigment in general, but chances are the pigment you need more of is yellow. Look at the tone of the color; is it too warm? Too cool? Too yellow? You can almost always tell by looking at yourself in a mirror in daylight with a makeup swatch on your cheek; you'll instantly see that the clean skin next to the makeup swatch is more red, more yellow, lighter, darker, or whatever.

- When blending makeup for dark skin tones you can reach a point where it just needs a certain richness or deepness that you can't quite nail down; this is a great place to add the tiniest amount of blue ultramarine. Try $\frac{1}{64}$ teaspoon or less—it will add an incredible depth of color.

- Once you start to get close to a final color blend, try it all over your entire face. Almost nobody's skin is completely uniform in color, so testing it on your cheek doesn't mean it'll be a perfect match on your forehead, and that's okay. Foundation is supposed to even out your skin tone, not cover it completely in a creepy masklike manner. Test your makeup all over, buff it in, and see what you think. Walk away from a mirror for a few minutes to let your mental image of yourself reset, and then see what you think again.

- If your face is dramatically lighter in the center than it is around the edges, you might want to blend up two foundations—one for the outside of your face, and one for the inside, blending the edges together when you apply them.

- Once you think you're done, start using your makeup on a daily basis. I've made batches that I think are a perfect match, only to decide they look just a touch too yellow 10 days later. No worries if this happens—take your notes from your first time and whip up a new batch or adjust the old one, dialing back or adding more of the color you think needs tweaking, tiptoeing forward until you find your new perfect combo (and remember to update your notes!). Sometimes I'll leave the makeup in the grinder for a few days and apply it from there before deciding if it's done or if it needs more fine-tuning.

- Don't be afraid to botch a batch. These ingredients are inexpensive, we're working with relatively small amounts, and that's how you learn!

AIRBRUSHING POWDERS

DESIGNED TO CREATE THE ILLUSION OF A SMOOTH, CLEAR COMPLEXION WITHOUT FULL COVERAGE, THESE lightweight powders are fantastic for casual daily wear. The idea for them came to me late one night as I was thinking about sericite mica. Sericite mica is a really neat ingredient. It's powdered aluminum potassium silicate, a naturally occurring mica. It's often used as a filler in cosmetics, and it also helps improve slip and adhesion. The property I was excited about that late night, though, was its ability to scatter and diffuse light, creating a bit of a blur effect around the skin. This optical illusion helps to disguise imperfections, reducing the appearance of fine lines and pores without covering them.

All this got me to thinking: What would a powder that was almost entirely sericite mica do? I pulled out my cosmetics coffee grinder and set to work. The resulting powder triggered a gleeful *squee* fit. When applied, it gives an airbrushed look while still letting freckles and other bits of you shine through. I find it's perfect for everyday wear, especially if you combine it with a bit of concealer (or well-behaved skin).

Because these airbrushing powders are just a blend of your Essential Mineral Makeup and sericite mica, you can easily make it in a variety of different strengths. More makeup and less mica makes for a higher-coverage powder; the more mica you use, the less coverage you'll get. The blends that use more sericite mica than mineral makeup include some extra oil to keep the powder creamy and prevent it from poufing out too much when you use it.

Once you're familiar with these blends, you can feel free to tweak the amounts of Essential Mineral Makeup and sericite mica based on how you like your airbrushing powder.

Airbrushing Powder

HIGH-COVERAGE AIRBRUSHING POWDER

1 teaspoon prepared Essential Mineral Makeup (page 84)

$^1/_2$ teaspoon sericite mica

MEDIUM-COVERAGE AIRBRUSHING POWDER

1 teaspoon prepared Essential Mineral Makeup (page 84)

1 teaspoon sericite mica

2 drops jojoba oil

LIGHT-COVERAGE AIRBRUSHING POWDER

1 teaspoon prepared Essential Mineral Makeup (page 84)

2 teaspoons sericite mica

4 drops jojoba oil

Since we'll be working with fine powders, start by putting on your dust mask. Next, choose an Airbrushing Powder blend and measure out the required amounts of Essential Mineral Makeup, sericite mica, and oil into your cosmetics-only coffee grinder. Place a sheet of plastic wrap between the grinder and the lid, and blend the powders together for about 20 seconds. Leave the powder to settle for at least 3 minutes before removing the lid, rapping it sharply with the back of a spoon to knock down any powder that might have crawled up the edge of the grinding dish. Give everything a stir with a small spoon to make sure the powders are evenly blended; some coffee grinders will leave a layer of powder untouched beneath the blades. If that's the case, turn everything over with your spoon and blend again for another 20 seconds. Repeat as needed until you have a uniform powder.

Once you've got a uniform powder, transfer it to a 1-ounce (28 g) jar fitted with a sifter top.

Because this makeup doesn't include any oil, we aren't concerned about microbial spoilage, but the oil in it can oxidize and go rancid. The Essential Mineral Makeup contains the antioxidant vitamin E, which will help delay oxidization, so you should get at least a year of shelf life out of your Airbrushing Powder, assuming it is stored somewhere cool and dry. If it starts to smell off (like crayons), that's a sign that the oils have gone rancid; chuck out your makeup and make a fresh batch.

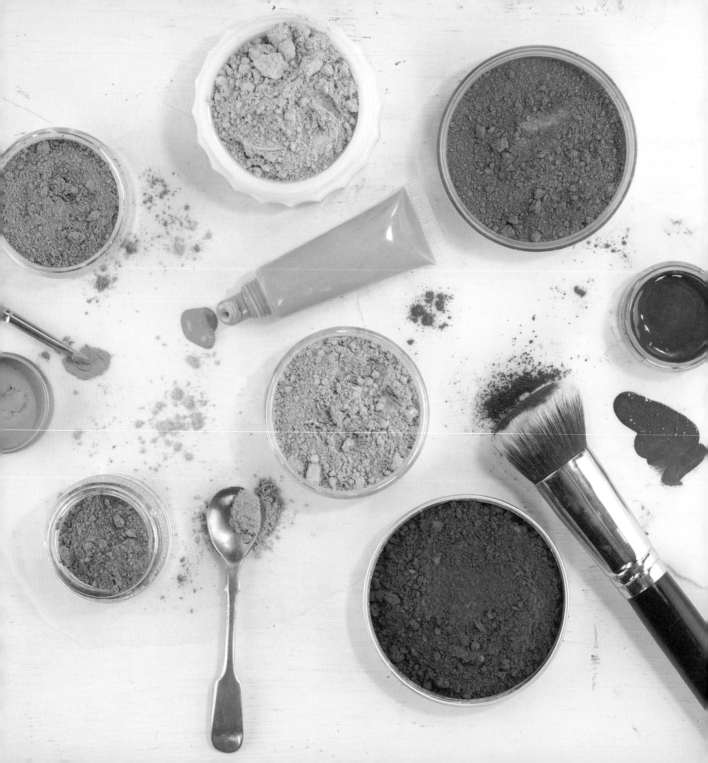

Essential Liquid Foundation

WHEN I'M TRYING TO RECREATE A COMMONLY AVAILABLE COSMETIC WITH AWESOME, NATURAL INGREDIENTS, the first thing I'll do is take a look at what's in the store-bought version, drop the icky stuff from the ingredients list, whip something up, and see how that works. It often works pretty well, but liquid foundation got the best of me for the longest time.

Liquid foundation is generally water-based, with pigments for color and opacity. Added to all that is a good dose of silicones to keep things silky smooth through application and wear, since powdered pigments and water dry out pretty quickly together, leaving you with something like face chalk. Ugh. So, my first attempts (many, many of them) were generally homemade lotion blended with mineral makeup. This resulted in failure after failure. I made many concoctions that looked like liquid foundation in the jar, but flat out didn't work. There would be no coverage, or it would be impossible to get even, smooth coverage. Some would pill on the face into eraser-shaving like clods that were none too flattering. Others would crack and crumble. One changed color drastically overnight and then sprouted mold in days. They were all awful.

So, I went back to the thing I was trying to recreate. I bought some liquid foundation, applied it, and had a bit of a revelation. A good, liquid foundation feels like argan oil on the skin when you apply it—a thin, smooth, liquid that you can glide across the skin. The cosmetics companies are using all those silicones, water, and isolated fatty acids so they can call their foundations "oil-free," but I'm not afraid of oil on my face. I like it. It's awesome. So, with that brain bug, I set off to try something new.

I started off by blending straight argan oil with mineral makeup, and that worked so well it felt a bit like cheating. But it works—brilliantly. It is easy to blend, sheers out beautifully, layers up wonderfully, stays on for ages, is crease-free, and is hydrating without being oily. You'll have to shake your jar or tube before application to keep everything distributed, but that's common with thinner liquid or serum foundations.

I like a kabuki brush for blending and buffing. Feel free to layer up in areas where you need additional coverage, and blend away. As with all cosmetics, this one looks best when applied to clean, dry, moisturized skin.

0.07 ounce (2 g) prepared
Essential Mineral Makeup
(page 84)

0.07 ounce (2 g) argan oil

2 drops vitamin E oil

Using your digital scale, weigh each ingredient out into a small container—0.17 fluid ounce (5 mL) is a great size for a pot, but you could also blend everything together in a small bowl and transfer it to a squeezable lip gloss tube for easy dispensing (you'll need to increase the batch size if you do this to fill the tube). Gently stir the Essential Mineral Makeup and oils together with a toothpick until you have a wee pot of smooth foundation (this will take about 1 minute). Voilà! This recipe can easily be scaled up; just be sure to keep a one-to-one by weight ratio between the powder and the oil.

As this foundation doesn't include any water, we aren't worried about microbial growth, but the argan oil in the foundation can oxidize and go rancid. The vitamin E will help prevent this, and you should get at least a year of shelf life if you store your foundation somewhere relatively cool and dry (though you'll likely use it all up well before then!). If you notice your foundation has started to smell like crayons or old nuts, that's a sign your argan oil has oxidized, so chuck it out and make a fresh batch.

Tip: You can also make this foundation using one of your Airbrushing Powders (page 91) instead of the full-strength Essential Mineral Makeup for a tinted moisturizer. I have found that pure sericite needs to be blended with more oil than Essential Mineral Makeup does, so you'll need to add some more argan oil (especially if you're using one of the lighter coverage powder blends that's mostly sericite mica).

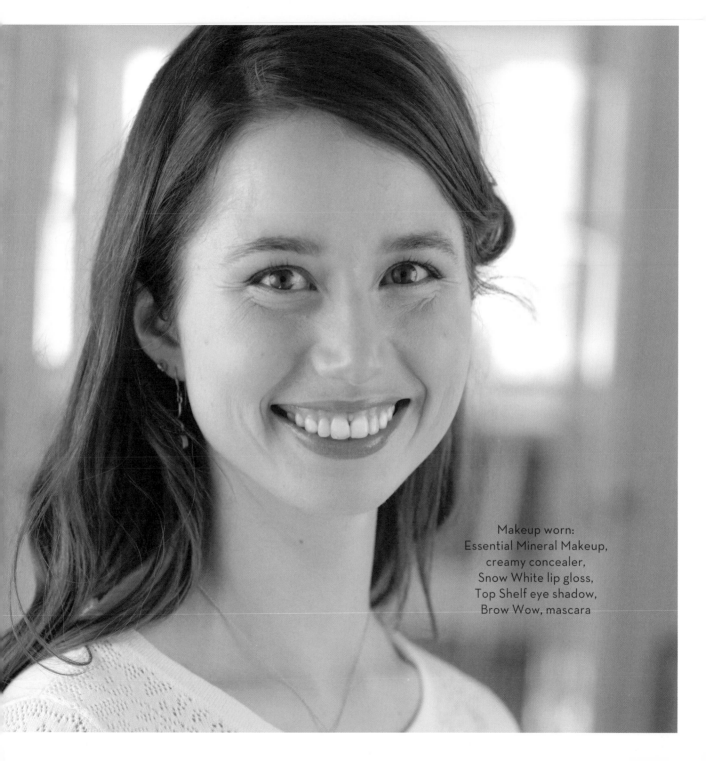

Makeup worn:
Essential Mineral Makeup,
creamy concealer,
Snow White lip gloss,
Top Shelf eye shadow,
Brow Wow, mascara

Creamy Concealer

THIS CREAMY, HIGHLY PIGMENTED CONCEALER IS FANTASTIC FOR COVERING UP BLEMISHES AND SHEERING out over areas that need a bit of extra coverage. It layers up beautifully, and since it's made with your Essential Mineral Makeup, it'll match your foundation. I've included some extra-healing vitamin E oil to help encourage blemishes to heal as well. Score!

0.03 ounce (1 g) refined beeswax

0.07 ounce (2 g) jojoba oil

0.1 ounce (3 g) prepared Essential Mineral Makeup (page 84)

5 drops vitamin E oil

Prepare a water bath by filling a small saucepan with approximately 2 inches (5 cm) of water and bringing it to a gentle simmer.

Using your digital scale, weigh the ingredients into a heat-resistant glass measuring cup and place that measuring cup in your water bath. Melt everything through, stirring to combine—this will take about 10 minutes. It's a good idea to use a thin, flexible silicone spatula to stir with, smearing it against the bottom of your measuring cup to ensure all the powder is thoroughly incorporating.

Once everything has melted together and the Essential Mineral Makeup is thoroughly blended into the melted oils, remove the measuring cup from the water bath and dry off the outside before pouring your concealer into a 0.17 ounce (5 g) tin. Leave it to solidify before using. It will only take about 10 minutes for your concealer to solidify enough to use, but it will continue to harden and thicken up for up to 24 hours after you pour it, so don't be surprised if it seems far too soft at first.

Because this concealer doesn't contain any water, we're only concerned about rancidity, which the vitamin E will help prevent. This concealer should last at least a year if kept dry and stored somewhere relatively cool. If you notice it's started to smell a bit like crayons or old nuts, that's a sign that the oils have oxidized and gone rancid; throw it away and make a fresh batch.

COLOR CORRECTION

If you enjoy poking about makeup shops, you've likely encountered facial palettes of rather peculiar colors; peachy oranges, lilac purples, and minty greens colors that look more at home at a baby shower or in a face paint palette than in a cosmetics store. These palettes are for color correcting; using complimentary colors to optically cancel out unwanted tones in our skin. Green neutralizes red, lavender neutralizes yellow (and yellow neutralizes purples), and orange helps neutralize blues. We can use this knowledge to easily create color-correcting variations of our concealer and foundation to tackle our individual needs.

As somebody with some red in her complexion, I'll make a half batch of my Essential Liquid Foundation (page 93) and stir in the smallest amount of green chromium oxide (just a few specks, really). I'm left with something that's not at all visibly green, but when I blend it into any redder areas of my face while I'm applying my foundation, the redness magically vanishes!

If you need a purple tint, try adding a wee bit of carmine and blue ultramarine to some foundation (or violet ultramarine, if you have it). For added orange, add a bit more red and yellow iron oxide.

If you'd prefer a creamy, sheer color-correcting base to work with before applying foundation over top, the Cream Base we use to make blush, bronzer, and highlighter (page 108) is a great place to start; simply mix in green oxide to cancel out red, a blend of blue ultramarine and carmine (for lavender), or a blend of yellow iron oxide and carmine (for orange). If you want a powder color corrector, the Powder Base (page 98) is perfectly suited; just blend it up and add whatever color you need to it. You'll be surprised at how little added color you need; $1/64$ or $1/32$ of a teaspoon is often more than enough to even out your coloring (too much yellow and you might find your purple under-eye circles start to look like patches of jaundice instead!).

Tip: I've found that some of the lipstick pigment blends make brilliant color correctors. For example, Blushing Taupe (page 168) is fantastic for canceling out under-eye circles in medium skin tones. Since the lipstick bases are a bit stiff for facial application, turn any lipstick color blend into a creamy color corrector by doubling the pigments and mixing them into a batch of the Cream Base (page 108).

Powder Base: Blush, Highlighter, and Bronzer

THIS SILKY POWDER BASE IS INCREDIBLY VERSATILE. THE BASE POWDER IS TRANSLUCENT AND LIGHTWEIGHT, and comes together in a jiffy in your cosmetics coffee grinder. From there we'll add some iron oxides and other pigments to create your perfect powdered highlighters, blushes, and bronzers!

MAKES APPROXIMATELY
0.21 OUNCE (6 G)

1 teaspoon sericite mica

1 teaspoon starch (arrowroot, wheat, or corn)

1 teaspoon white kaolin clay

1/16 teaspoon magnesium stearate

1/8 teaspoon titanium dioxide

10 drops jojoba oil

4 drops vitamin E oil

Pigment (see Color Blends sections on pages 100 [blush], 102 [highlighter], and 104 [bronzer])

Grab your dust mask. Since we're dealing with fine powders, you need to wear a dust mask so you don't inhale them.

Measure the sericite mica, starch, clay, magnesium stearate, titanium dioxide, jojoba oil, and vitamin E oil out into your coffee grinder and lay a sheet of plastic wrap over the grinder before popping the lid on, sandwiching the cling film between the grinder and the lid. Blend everything together to a fine, uniform powder; about 20 seconds. Sharply rap the lid of the grinder with the back of a spoon to knock the powder down into the grinding dish and let the dust settle for at least 3 minutes before removing the lid. Give the powder a stir—many coffee grinders will leave a layer of untouched powder in the dish beneath the blades, so you'll want to get in there with a spoon and ensure everything is turned over before giving it another blend or two.

Now it's time to start adding pigment!

Once your powder base is thoroughly blended, it's time to add your pigments and turn it into blush, bronzer, or highlighter—your imagination is the limit! Just add pigments and/or micas and blend until everything is thoroughly uniform; at least 20 seconds (remember to stir down to the bottom of the dish between blending sessions to ensure no powder is getting left behind), and you're done. I've developed quite a few color blends to get you started, but feel free to strike out on your own as well! If you aren't sure about one of my color blends, work up to it, using a makeup brush to test the powder on your face as you go,

you may n dioxide ll for, and a blush or er powder add more mmer, add so you can it, transfer smetic jar

Because these powders are almost entirely dry inorganic minerals, the only spoilage we're concerned about is the jojoba oil oxidizing and going rancid, but the vitamin E (which is an antioxidant) will help prevent that. These powders should last for at least a year stored in a relatively cool, dry place. If you start to notice your powder smells off (like crayons or old nuts), that's a sign the oil has oxidized, and it's time to throw out your powder and make a fresh batch.

Tip: Grinding colored micas (like silver, gold, bronze, and copper) can separate the color from the shimmer, dulling the overall effect in your final powder. If you want maximum shimmer, stir your colored micas into powdered cosmetics after you've finished grinding everything else together; micas are light enough that they don't need to be ground up to incorporate reasonably well.

POWDER BLUSH COLOR BLENDS

A powder blush is a beautifully simple thing to make, and fantastically simple to customize. We'll start with our powder base and color it from there. More intense or less? We can do that. Pink, red, coral, or peach? Not a problem. Shimmer or no shimmer? Done deal. Bring on the blush! I've found $3/64$ of a teaspoon of pigment in the powder base is a great place to start for a blush, though this really is just a guideline, as some pigments pop more on the skin than others, and some skin tones need more pigment than others. If you find your blush isn't pigmented enough for you, simply increase the pigments as needed, blending and testing between additions.

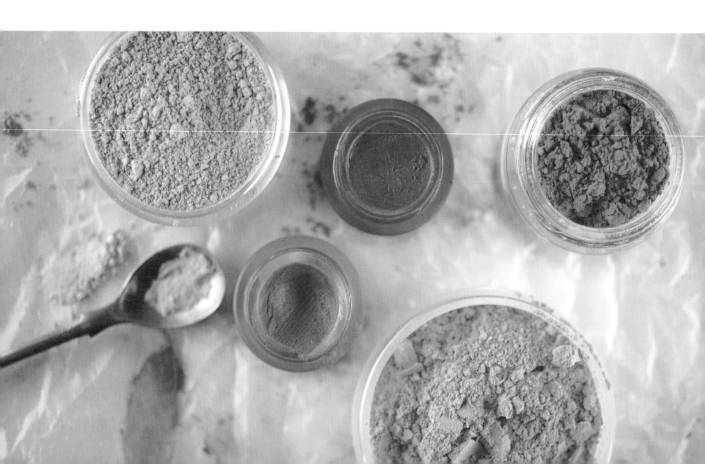

Elle Woods Blush

A SURPRISINGLY WEARABLE POPPING PINK BLUSH, PERFECT FOR A FRESH, SPRINGY GLOW.

1 recipe Powder Base, prepared (page 98)

$3/64$ teaspoon carmine

$1/32$ teaspoon silver mica

Summer Dusk Blush

A SOFTER, LESS PIGMENTED PINK THAT BUILDS UP TO NATURAL GLOW BEAUTIFULLY.
Because this blush is fairly low pigment, it's great for really pale skin, but you'll
want to double (or even triple) the pigments for darker skin.

1 recipe Powder Base, prepared (page 98)

$3/64$ teaspoon yellow iron oxide

$3/128$ teaspoon carmine

Deep Coral Blush

A FANTASTIC, ALL-PURPOSE EARTHY-RED BLUSH
that looks wonderful on a wide variety of complexions.

1 recipe Powder Base, prepared (page 98)

$3/64$ teaspoon red iron oxide

Teensy speck blue ultramarine

POWDER HIGHLIGHTER COLOR BLENDS

WHEN IT COMES TO HIGHLIGHTING, THERE ARE TWO STRATEGIES FOR REFLECTING LIGHT; WITH SOMEthing lighter than the skin around it, or something shimmery, like a mica (or both!). Titanium dioxide is usually that lighter ingredient—since it's bright white, it's guaranteed to be lighter than your skin. We don't want to use too much titanium dioxide, though, or you'll end up with a powder so strong that it's hard to use without ending up entirely too pale. The amount of titanium dioxide that's right for you will depend on your skin tone; darker skin needs less, paler skin needs more. The amount of mica you'll use is entirely dependent on your taste for shimmer. Always start with less than the recipe calls for and work up, testing between additions and taking notes, until you find exactly what you're looking for.

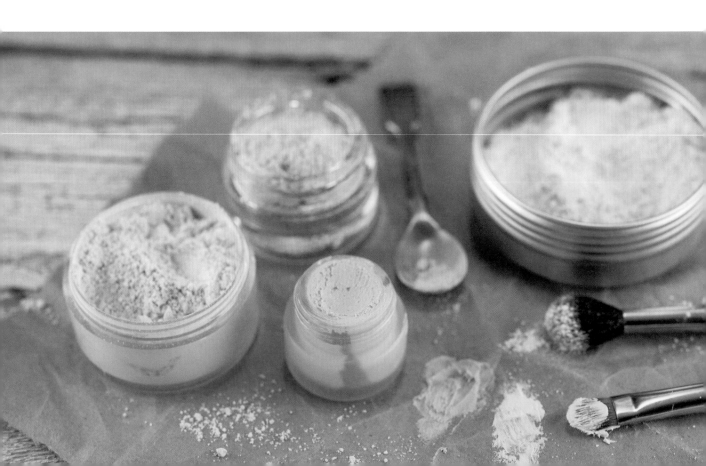

Fairy Dust Highlighting Powder

FAIRY DUST IS A BRIGHT WHITE, SHIMMERY HIGHLIGHT THAT'S REMINISCENT OF TINKERBELL'S fairy dust. While it won't make you fly, it'll lift your brow bones beautifully.

1 recipe Powder Base, prepared (page 98)

1 teaspoon titanium dioxide

$5/_{32}$ teaspoon silver mica

Gold Dust Highlighting Powder

THIS SOFT YELLOW POWDER HAS A LOVELY GOLDEN GLOW THAT'S BEAUTIFUL ON WARMER SKIN TONES.

1 recipe Powder Base, prepared (page 98)

$1/_{16}$ teaspoon yellow iron oxide

$1/_{16}$ teaspoon gold mica

Pink Satin Highlighting Powder

PERK UP CHEEKBONES WITH THIS SOFT PINK, lightly shimmery powder; it's great for fair skin tones.

1 recipe Powder Base, prepared (page 98)

$1/_2$ teaspoon titanium dioxide

$1/_{128}$ teaspoon carmine

$1/_{32}$ teaspoon silver mica

POWDER BRONZER COLOR BLENDS

THESE BRONZERS BRING THE SUN TO YOU WITH WARM, BRONZED TONES THAT LEAVE YOU LOOKING BEAUtifully sun-kissed (they're also fantastic for contouring). You can choose to go full shimmer, stay matte, or work with something in between. If you're quite fair, you'll appreciate the ability to work the color up to something that looks like a bronzer rather than a dirt smudge on your complexion. If you're darker, you'll find these bronzers can make lovely highlighters, and you can increase the pigment to make a high impact bronzer that's perfect for you. As always, work up to your final blend, testing between additions and taking notes so you can always recreate your perfect bronzer.

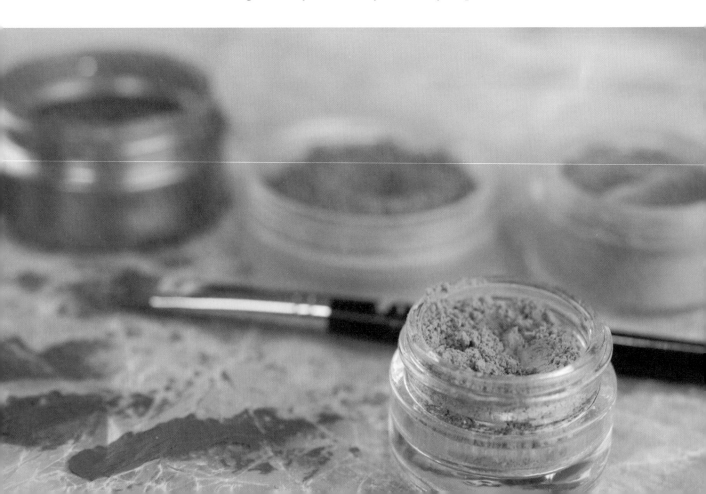

Tawny Glimmer

A FANTASTIC WARM BRONZE SHADE WITH JUST A HINT OF SHIMMER—
I find it works beautifully on a wide variety of skin tones and layers up beautifully.

1 recipe Powder Base, prepared (page 98) $^1/_{16}$ teaspoon yellow iron oxide
$^3/_{64}$ teaspoon brown iron oxide $^1/_{32}$ teaspoon bronze mica
$^1/_{32}$ teaspoon red iron oxide

Australian Gold Rush

THIS WARM BRONZER PACKS A WONDERFUL SHIMMERY PUNCH, THANKS TO A BLEND OF
three different micas (though you can feel free to just use one if that's what you have on hand).
It's great for bronzing medium skin tones, and makes a fantastic highlight for dark skin tones.

1 recipe Powder Base, prepared (page 98) $^1/_{16}$ teaspoon bronze mica
$^1/_{16}$ teaspoon brown iron oxide $^1/_{32}$ teaspoon gold mica
$^1/_{16}$ teaspoon yellow iron oxide $^1/_{32}$ teaspoon copper mica
$^1/_{32}$ teaspoon red iron oxide

Playa Kiss

PLAYA KISS IS A GREAT MATTE BRONZER AND CONTOUR POWDER FOR PALER COMPLEXIONS,
as it's not too heavily pigmented. If you're darker, feel free to double (or even triple)
the pigments to make a bronzer that works for you.

1 recipe Powder Base, prepared (page 98)
$^1/_{64}$ teaspoon brown iron oxide
$^3/_{32}$ teaspoon yellow iron oxide

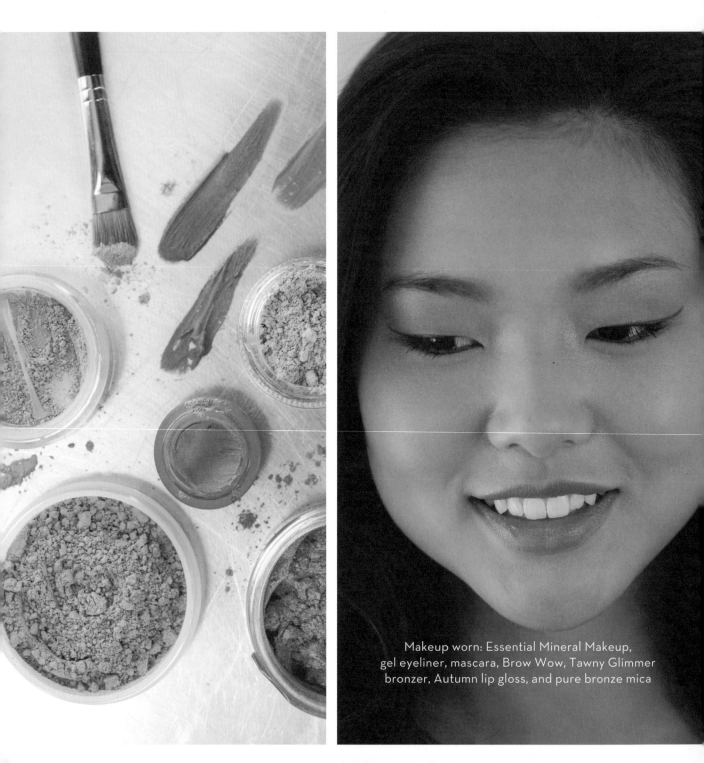

Makeup worn: Essential Mineral Makeup, gel eyeliner, mascara, Brow Wow, Tawny Glimmer bronzer, Autumn lip gloss, and pure bronze mica

DO YOU PREFER PRESSED POWDERS OVER LOOSE?

No worries, that's easy to do with ingredients we already have! Once your powder is done, weigh it out, and add more magnesium stearate until your powder is approximately 10 percent magnesium stearate by weight. These finished powdered highlighters, blushes, and bronzers weigh about 0.28 ounce (8 g), so you'd want to add approximately 0.03 ounce (1 g) of magnesium stearate and blend that all together in your coffee grinder (remember to wear your dust mask!) with a few extra drops of jojoba oil (approximately one extra drop for every 0.07 [2 g] of powder). You're aiming for a uniform powder that looks a bit like biscuit dough; crumbly and easy to press together. Once you've got a clumpy powder, it's time to start pressing!

To press a powder, you'll need something to press the powder into (I love picking up empty vintage makeup compacts at antique shops), something to press it with, and a bit of parchment paper or plastic wrap to go between the powder and the presser (I prefer parchment, but if you're pressing into the base of something quite deep, the flexibility of cling film is nice). You can purchase pressing tools that look like a quarter with a little knob attached, but a clean coin, a round bottle cap, the base of a shot glass, or the back of a relatively flat spoon will do the trick—you really just need something flat that you can use to stamp the powder down.

Spoon a bit of the powder into your compact, doing your best to scatter it around evenly, and then lay a piece of parchment paper over top and press that powder down, gently at first, and increasing pressure as you go. As the powder compacts down, add more from the coffee grinder, taking care to cover the edges and corners of the compact and press it all down firmly. You'll be surprised by how much powder you can pack into a fairly small space!

Once you've filled your compact, you're done. If you want to add a bit of a professional touch you can place a small piece of woven fabric over the powder and do another pressing with that in place for a subtle textured look.

You can do this with any of the cosmetic powders in the book, just be sure to recalculate the amount of magnesium stearate required based on the weight of the powder you're using. The formula for that is pretty simple: Multiply the weight of the powder by 100, and then divide that number by 90. That will give you the desired total weight of the original powder plus the magnesium stearate, so simply subtract the weight of the original powder to get the amount of magnesium stearate you need to add. For 8 g of powder that would look like: 8 g × 100 = 800. 800 ÷ 90 = 8.88 g. 8.88 g – 8 g (the weight of the starter powder) = 0.88 g, which we'll round to 0.9 g, and that's how much magnesium stearate you would add.

Cream Base: Blush, Highlighter, and Bronzer

IF YOU LIKE YOUR BLUSH, HIGHLIGHTER, OR BRONZER IN CREAMY FORM, YOU'LL BE THRILLED TO FIND OUT it's just as easy (maybe even easier) as making the powdered versions. We'll start with a simple, four-ingredient cream base, and then add pigments and micas to transform it into wonderful wee pots of creamy, colorful fun that make brilliant tinted lip balms as well.

MAKES APPROXIMATELY
0.35 OUNCE (10 G)

0.1 ounce (3 g) refined beeswax

0.21 ounce (6 g) jojoba oil

10 drops vitamin E oil

¼ teaspoon magnesium stearate

Pigment (see Color Blends sections on pages 110 [blush], 111 [highlighter], and 112 [bronzer])

Measure the beeswax, jojoba oil, vitamin E oil, and magnesium stearate into a small saucepan and stir everything together with a flexible silicone spatula, taking care to break up the clumps of magnesium stearate so it will melt nicely. Place the saucepan on the stove over low heat to melt everything together. The reason we're melting this base over direct heat instead of using a water bath is because the magnesium stearate has a high enough melting point (190°F [88°C]) that melting it in a water bath is quite difficult and time-consuming. Keep an eye on the melting oils so they don't scorch, stirring the mixture as it melts to help speed things along. Remove the pan from the heat as soon as everything has melted and the mixture is uniform and transparent (unmelted magnesium stearate will make the otherwise melted liquid look cloudy; you're not done melting until the liquid is clear). As this recipe is fairly small, it will only take 5 to 10 minutes to melt over low heat. If the base overheats, it will scorch and you'll find the final product looks oddly curdled once you add the pigments (it'll also smell funny).

Now it's time to start adding pigment!

I recommend transferring the cream base to a small bowl (something that holds about half a cup [125 mL]) for this part;

it makes for easier color blending and allows you to easily pop the bowl into a hot water bath to melt the base again if it sets up on you as you're working. The smaller bowl also makes for much faster cleanup.

When it comes to blending powdered pigments into a cream base (this goes for lipsticks as well), a flexible silicone spatula is your best friend. Use it to break up clumps and smear the pigments against the bottom and sides of the dish to blend everything together. You'll see streaks of distinct pigments across the bottom of the dish as you drag your spatula across it; after 3 to 5 minutes of blending those should virtually disappear, and that's when you're done. If you're confident in your color blend and feel like going the extra mile, it's really helpful to give your pigments a quick blitz in your coffee grinder. Remember to sandwich a piece of plastic wrap between the grinder and the lid so you don't lose a lot of pigment to the inside of the coffee grinder. After you've ground your pigments together for a solid 20 to 30 seconds, add your color blend to your cream base and proceed as usual. Take care to get as much pigment as possible out of the grinder and into your cream base (a small, fluffy, cosmetic brush is really helpful) so you don't end up with a noticeably weaker color blend in your finished product. If the cream base starts to solidify before you're done stirring in your pigments, just set the bowl in a shallow pan of steaming hot water to loosen everything back up and keep on blending.

Be sure to test your concoction on your face as you go, blending it in as you would in daily use. If you're quite dark-skinned, you'll want to err on the side of caution with titanium dioxide in highlighters to avoid looking ashy, and if you're quite fair-skinned, you'll want to be tentative with the pigments in cream bronzer to avoid looking dirty.

Once you're done blending in the pigments, pour your creamy concoction into a 0.35-ounce (10 g) jar and leave it to set up before using. It'll solidify enough to use in about 10 minutes, but it will continue to harden for up to 24 hours after you pour it, so don't worry if it seems a bit soft at first.

Because there's no water in these creamy cosmetics, we aren't concerned about microbial spoilage. The oils will eventually oxidize and go rancid, but the vitamin E in the recipe will help delay that. You should get a shelf life of at least a year if you store your cosmetics somewhere relatively cool and dry. If you notice any of your creamy cosmetics have started to smell like crayons or old nuts, chuck it and make a new batch—that's a sign that the oils have oxidized.

CREAM BLUSH COLOR BLENDS

THESE WEE POTS OF CREAMY PINK AND RED BLEND INTO THE SKIN BEAUTIFULLY, PERKING UP YOUR CHEEKS and doubling as fantastic tinted lip balms.

1985

THIS BRIGHT PINK BLUSH BLENDS IN BEAUTIFULLY FOR A
soft pink glow, or can be layered up to create a great '80s look.

1 recipe Cream Base, prepared (page 108) | $3/64$ teaspoon carmine
$1/32$ teaspoon titanium dioxide | $1/32$ teaspoon silver mica

Dusty Cranberry

A COOLER RUDDY-RED BLUSH THAT WORKS WELL ALL YEAR,
but is especially well suited to fall and winter wear.

1 recipe Cream Base, prepared (page 108) | $1/32$ teaspoon carmine
$1/32$ teaspoon titanium dioxide | $1/16$ teaspoon silver mica
$1/16$ teaspoon red iron oxide

CREATE YOUR OWN

If you want to make your own color blends, I've found that $3/16$ of a teaspoon of pigment is a good place to start, though you can always use less if you're quite fair and more if you're quite dark.

CREAM HIGHLIGHTER COLOR BLENDS

ELEVATE CHEEKBONES AND CREATE DEPTH WITH BRIGHT AND CREAMY HIGHLIGHTERS. TRY ADDING MORE mica for extra shimmer, and feel free to tweak the amount of titanium dioxide, using more for paler complexions and less for darker skin tones.

Brightlighter

THIS CREAMY COOL PINK HIGHLIGHT IS BRILLIANT ON MANY COMPLEXIONS
and works beautifully to open up the eyes when used on the brow bone and inner eye.

1 recipe Cream Base, prepared (page 108)

$^1/_4$ teaspoon titanium dioxide

$^1/_8$ teaspoon sericite mica

$^1/_{16}$ teaspoon silver mica

Teensy speck carmine

White Opal

STEP UP THE SHIMMER WITH THIS BRIGHT
white highlighter that's brilliant on cheekbones.

1 recipe Cream Base, prepared (page 108)

$^3/_8$ teaspoon titanium dioxide

$^1/_4$ teaspoon silver mica

$^1/_8$ teaspoon sericite mica

CREATE YOUR OWN

Check out the lipstick color blends on page 167. They're designed to turn 0.17 ounce (5 g) of lipstick base into lipstick. One recipe of the Cream Base makes approximately 0.33 ounce (10 g), so if you add the pigment blend for one lipstick, you'll have a creamy concoction that's roughly half the pigment strength of lipstick.

CREAM BRONZER COLOR BLENDS

EMBRACE A SUNNY GLOW WITH THESE CREAMY, BEACHY BRONZERS. DEPENDING ON YOUR TASTE FOR shimmer you can use more or less mica, and feel free to experiment with copper and gold as an alternative to bronze if you're feeling inspired!

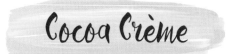

Penny Glow

WARM AND A BIT COPPERY, THIS BRONZER LENDS A SOFT SUN-KISSED
tone with just a hint of red (try it as a bronzed blush in the summer!).

1 recipe Cream Base, prepared (page 108) | $1/_{32}$ teaspoon yellow iron oxide
$1/_{32}$ teaspoon titanium dioxide | $1/_{64}$ teaspoon red iron oxide
$1/_{64}$ teaspoon brown iron oxide | $1/_{32}$ teaspoon bronze mica

Cocoa Crème

PURE BROWN WITH A HINT OF SHIMMER, THIS BRONZER BLENDS OUT BEAUTIFULLY
on most complexions (though darker skin tones will need more brown oxide).

1 recipe Cream Base, prepared (page 108)
$1/_{64}$ teaspoon brown oxide
$1/_{32}$ teaspoon bronze mica

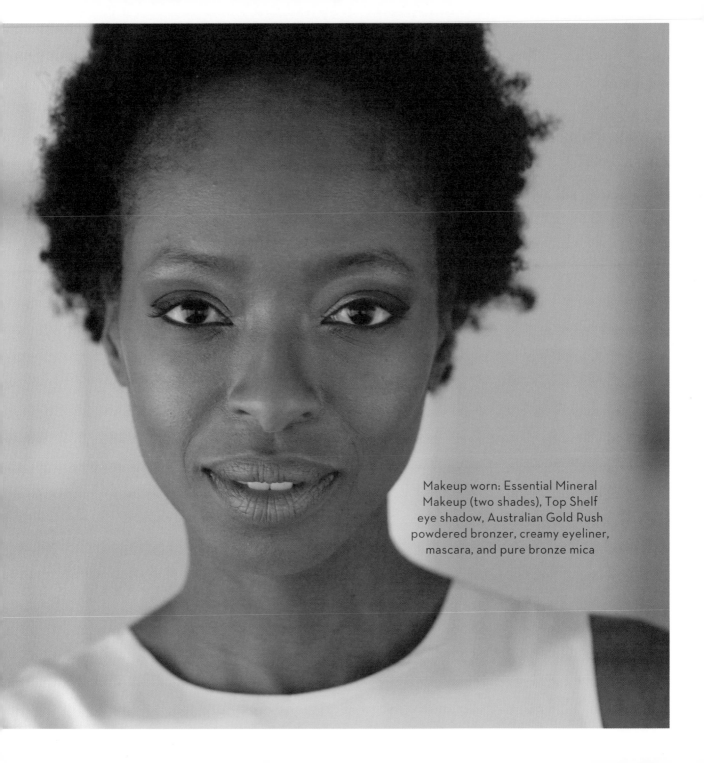

Makeup worn: Essential Mineral Makeup (two shades), Top Shelf eye shadow, Australian Gold Rush powdered bronzer, creamy eyeliner, mascara, and pure bronze mica

Matte Anti-Shine and Setting Powder

THIS CLAY-POWERED TRANSLUCENT POWDER IS JUST THE THING FOR SETTING MAKEUP AND COMBATING shine. A light dusting will do the trick, absorbing excess oil to leave you looking flawless. Despite its white appearance it vanishes on dark and light skin tones alike, taking any shiny patches with it.

MAKES ABOUT 4 TEASPOONS

2 teaspoons starch (arrowroot, wheat, or corn)

2 teaspoons white kaolin clay

¼ teaspoon calcium carbonate

5 drops jojoba oil

3 drops vitamin E oil

Start by putting on your dust mask as we're working with fine powders. Measure everything into your coffee grinder, sandwich a piece of plastic wrap between the grinder and the lid, and blend everything together for 20 seconds. Rap the lid of the grinder sharply with the back of a spoon to knock down any powder that has crawled up the edge of the grinding dish, and leave the lid on for at least 3 minutes after grinding to allow the powder to settle. Once you remove the lid, be sure to stir the powder around in the coffee grinder to ensure everything is thoroughly blended as some coffee grinders will leave a layer of untouched powder beneath the blade—turning everything over with a spoon and giving the lot another buzz in the coffee grinder will solve that!

To use, transfer the powder to a 1-ounce (28 g) jar fitted with a sifter lid. Use a large powder brush to dust it over your skin to set your makeup after application, and throughout the day to erase shine. I don't recommend pressing this powder as it works best when it's light and fluffy.

Because this powder is mostly made from inorganic materials and contains no water, the only type of spoilage we're concerned about is the jojoba oil going rancid, which the vitamin E will help prevent. This powder should last at least a year if stored somewhere reasonably cool and dry. If it starts to smell like crayons, that's a sign that the jojoba oil has oxidized and means it's time to throw out your setting powder and make a fresh batch.

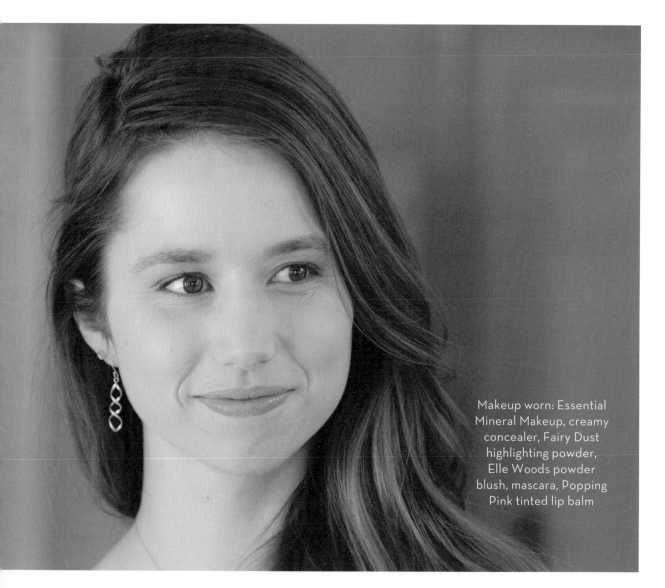

Makeup worn: Essential Mineral Makeup, creamy concealer, Fairy Dust highlighting powder, Elle Woods powder blush, mascara, Popping Pink tinted lip balm

CHAPTER FIVE

EYE MAKEUP

I love eye makeup. It was my first cosmetic love, starting with poorly applied blue eye shadow and moving onward to winged liner and smoky eyes. Well done eye makeup can completely transform a face, and there's so much room to play. While we're generally limited to a fairly narrow color palette for lips and the face, you can confidently break out the entire rainbow when it comes to your eye makeup, making homemade eye makeup extra awesome. If you want eyeliner in every color under the sun, it's yours!

Rainbow fun aside, eye makeup is tricky to formulate. All that blinking we do makes adhesion a challenge—eye shadows and eyeliners smudge and crawl into creases, turning your carefully blended smoky eye into an accidental panda. Oily eyelids complicate adhesion further, causing colors to slip and slide up to your brows and clump in creases. Sensitive eyes limit the ingredients we can use so you don't end up feeling like your eyes are on fire, and sensitive skin means we need soft, creamy powders and pencils more than anywhere else. Unfortunately, soft and creamy and amazing adhesion don't usually go together, and there lies the challenge.

The recipes in this chapter have been obsessively developed and carefully tested. I've recruited coworkers and friends for help, and I'm confident that these recipes will work for you. The ingredients I've included, while sometimes a bit strange, are necessary for awesome performance. *Tip:* Nothing in this chapter is waterproof, so don't tightline with the eyeliners and avoid getting anything in your waterline (like mascara)—you'll find that's rather itchy until you blink it out!

EYE PRIMER

Out of all the recipes in the book, this one proved to be the most problematic. Testing various formulas saw me leaving the house with impeccable eye makeup, only to return hours later looking like I'd applied my eyeliner with both my eyes shut. I easily tested upward of forty different formulas, leaving my kitchen littered with dishes of various pastes, powders, and goos for months on end.

Oil from our skin is what causes our eye

makeup to do the moonwalk up and down our eyelids, accumulating in clumpy lines and smudging up into the socket. Commercial primers tend to fight oil by using synthetic silicones and other film-forming ingredients to create a barrier between your oil-creating skin and your eye makeup, but since we're not using silicones, this primer goes the absorption route instead. Several of the ingredients we're using in this book are fantastic oil absorbers—both calcium carbonate and bentonite clay are amazingly powerful oil-absorbing ingredients, and I found they made primers that performed really well. Unfortunately, they both have pH levels around 9, and primers made with them left my eyeballs feeling like they were on fire (though my eyeliner was impeccable all day!). Lowering the pH with the addition of an acid also lowered the oil-absorbing abilities of both ingredients, so I eventually abandoned those ingredients.

After more research, more experimenting, and many more days of my eyeliner migrating all over my face, I pulled out a bag of silica microspheres and decided to give them a try. Silicon dioxide is highly absorbent (you've probably found little packets of it as silica gel in your shoe boxes to help keep your shoes dry during transport and storage), and in microsphere format it's silky smooth. Applied straight to the skin it worked really well; almost too well! I could feel my eyelids drying out for the first hour after application, but my eyeliner stayed put for hours. From there I developed two different silica microsphere powered primers to keep my eye makeup in place, both of which are delightfully simple and crazy effective.

Silica microspheres are one of the more expensive powders we're using, but thankfully we won't need much. A teaspoon of silica microspheres weighs about 0.07 ounce (2 g), and that's enough for *a lot* of primer. If you can purchase 0.35 ounce (10 g) or less that'll be more than enough.

Tip: Despite the similar names, the silica microspheres we're using are very different from silicones like dimethicone, which are synthetic polymers that contain silicon.

Powdered Eye Primer

THIS SIMPLE APPROACH IS BEST SUITED FOR OILIER EYELIDS, OR IF YOU'RE PRESERVATIVE-AVERSE. MY TESTS easily got upward of 12 hours of great wear with it (even overnight wear is pretty awesome)! This one works beautifully if you're planning on wearing Creamy Eyeliner (page 128) or Gel Eyeliner (page 133) without eye shadow, but it's also fantastic with eye shadow, preventing creasing all day.

⅛ teaspoon silica microspheres

1 recipe Essential Mineral Makeup, prepared (page 84)

Put on your dust mask and measure the silica microspheres out into a small sifter jar—0.17 ounce (5 g) is a great size. The measurement honestly doesn't matter at all, we just want the silica microspheres to be in a convenient container with a sifter to help you apply it in tiny amounts and avoid inhaling it.

To prime your eyes, simply apply some of your Essential Mineral Makeup to dry, clean eyelids using a dense eye shadow brush, and then use a fluffy eye shadow brush to dust overtop of it with a tiny amount of silica microspheres. Wait 5 minutes for everything to set, and now you can apply your eye makeup! If you have extra-oily eyelids, dust overtop of your finished look with some more silica microspheres (I also find this extra coat of silica to be helpful if you're only applying Creamy Eyeliner [page 128]).

Because this is really just straight silica microspheres we aren't worried about spoilage as long as you keep them dry.

Tip: Even though the silica microspheres are really tiny, they're still irritating if they get into your eyes, just like any powder is. To prevent itchy eyes, take care not to apply too much silica when you're dusting it on—it's potent stuff, you don't need much.

Gel Eye Primer

IF YOU PREFER YOUR PRIMER TO HAVE A TRANSLUCENT FINISH, THIS GEL PRIMER IS FOR YOU. IT'S NOT AS powerful as the powdered primer, but my tests still got at least 10 hours of great wear with it.

$1/16$ teaspoon silica microspheres

10 drops water

3 drops vegetable glycerin

Broad-spectrum preservative (follow manufacturer's recommendation for usage amount; if your preservative is liquid, one drop will be more than enough)

Put on your dust mask and measure the silica microspheres, water, and vegetable glycerin out into a small jar—0.17 ounce (5 g) is a great size. Stir everything together with a toothpick until you have a uniform mixture (this will take about 1 minute), and you're done!

The silica microspheres will settle out of the liquids, so shake the jar before use to ensure everything is evenly mixed. Apply a small amount (about a drop) to each eyelid with a concealer brush, dust your lids with some extra silica microspheres, and let everything dry for 5 minutes before applying your eye makeup. For extra staying power, dust over your finished look with more silica microspheres.

Because this primer contains water, we need to include a broad-spectrum preservative to ward off microbial spoilage. Do not skip it—you don't want to get an eye infection from your primer! We're making this in small amounts to increase the chances of you using it all up before you notice any signs of spoilage, but if you happen to notice any changes in color, scent, or texture, chuck it out and make more.

Tip: Make sure you store this primer in a sealed container; depending on the humidity level where you live it can dry out or absorb extra moisture quite quickly!

EYE SHADOW

AFTER LIP GLOSS, EYE SHADOW WAS THE FIRST COSMETIC I EVER TRIED. I REMEMBER FINDING A WEE BLACK compact of sparkly "periwinkle" eye shadow in a grab bag of miscellaneous girly stuff from a nearby shop when I was about eleven and quickly deciding it was the prettiest color in the world. It was a sort of dusty blue-purple shade with a hefty dose of sparkle, and as soon as my mother would let me, I proudly rocked periwinkle finger-smudged eyelids at school along with my braces.

Over the years my taste in colors has shifted and my application methods have improved, but I still love a good eye shadow palette. I *especially* love a palette that's exactly what I want it to be. When we talk about the things we want in an eye shadow, there are definitely a few all-important characteristics. For starters, it should be available in all kinds of colors, and in a variety of pigment levels, depending on your preferences and skin tone. It should feel velvety and smooth when you apply it. It should blend beautifully and lend itself to precise application when needed. And then, when you're done applying it, it should stay where you put it and not go climbing into creases or looking to summit your brow bone every time you blink. This seems like a fairly short to-do list, but it can be a tricky one to complete.

My eye shadow base is soft and light, and applies very nearly sheer on even the darkest of skin. It can easily be colored, from light tints to deep, dark colors. It takes shimmer nicely, and feels like satin when you apply it. You can easily mix up a big batch of the base and keep it on hand, blending up a new color or two as needed. The bulk of the powder base is sheer sericite mica and silky arrowroot starch, with some added magnesium stearate for adhesion and slip. The boron nitride really is the magic maker here, taking our eye shadows from "meh" to "ooooooh," even in fairly small amounts. Boron nitride brings incredible creaminess and adhesion, and I have found it to be indispensable for truly wonderful homemade eye shadows. Last but not least, some calcium carbonate prolongs the wear of this eye shadow. Crease-free wear time without primer varies by the color of the eye shadow (more pigment lowers the wear time) and by the wearer's eyes; I can get 8 hours of crease-free wear with lighter colors, while some testers couldn't get 4. Anyhow, if you pair this eye shadow with my Powdered Eye Primer (page 118) or Gel Eye Primer (page 119), it'll go all day (and with the Powdered version, all night!) without creasing.

Because our base is sheer, the amount of pigment you add is really up to you and your skin tone. If you're quite pale, you'll find fairly small amounts of pigment produce eye shadows that really pop on your skin, and the darker your skin is, the more pigment you'll need.

Eye Shadow Powder Base

MAKES APPROXIMATELY 0.38 OUNCE (11 G)

2 teaspoons sericite mica

2 teaspoons arrowroot starch

$^3/_8$ teaspoon boron nitride

$^1/_8$ teaspoon magnesium stearate

$^1/_8$ teaspoon magnesium myristate

$^5/_{32}$ teaspoon calcium carbonate

35 drops jojoba oil

7 drops vitamin E oil

Pigment (see Color Palette Blends section on page 124)

To make your eye shadow base, start by grabbing your dust mask since we'll be whirring up fine powders and you don't want to inhale them. Measure all the powdered ingredients into your cosmetics-only coffee grinder and sandwich a piece of plastic wrap between the grinder and the lid. Blend everything together for about 20 seconds, leaving the lid on the grinder for a few minutes afterward to let the dust settle. Before removing the lid, rap it sharply with the back of a spoon to knock the powder back down in the grinding dish—it has a tendency to creep upward. Use a spoon to stir the powder around, checking to make sure there isn't a layer of untouched powder beneath the grinder blades. If there is, turn the powder over with your spoon and give everything another whir to ensure the base is thoroughly blended.

Up next: scatter the drops of jojoba oil and vitamin E oil over the powder and blend those in. This will probably require at least two blends as the oils have a tendency to drop down to the bottom of the grinding dish rather than incorporating at first, so you'll need to get in there with a spoon, scrape them up, and blend it all again.

Once you've got a uniform powder, that's it—eye shadow base! Transfer it to a jar and label it, and you're ready to start adding pigments to create your own rainbow of eye shadows.

Now it's time to start adding pigment!

In this book I provide three color palette blends to get you started. For each color simply measure 2 teaspoons of the eye shadow base (lightly spooned and leveled off; don't pack your measuring spoon) and the pigments listed into your coffee grinder and blend until you have a uniform eye shadow. Be sure to have a piece of plastic wrap sandwiched between the coffee grinder and the lid to reduce the volume of your grinder—this will make achieving a thorough and even color blend much easier. You'll need to scrape down the edges of your grinder between blendings to ensure you get everything worked in properly, and make sure you do at least two or three 20-second blends. When your eye shadow is thoroughly blended, scrape it into a 0.35 ounce (10 g) sifter jar and it's ready to use! Clean your coffee grinder between colors by running a tablespoon of rice through it and dusting it out with a small powder brush (grab a new piece of cling film, too).

Tip: Do you have extra-oily eyelids? Try adding another $1/32$ teaspoon of calcium carbonate to the eye shadow base to help absorb extra oil.

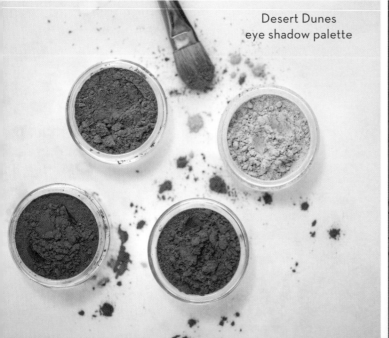

Desert Dunes
eye shadow palette

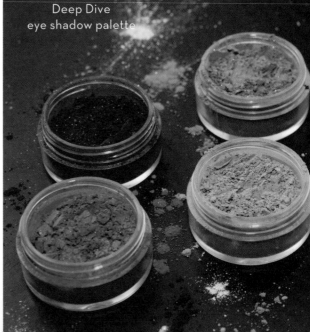

Deep Dive
eye shadow palette

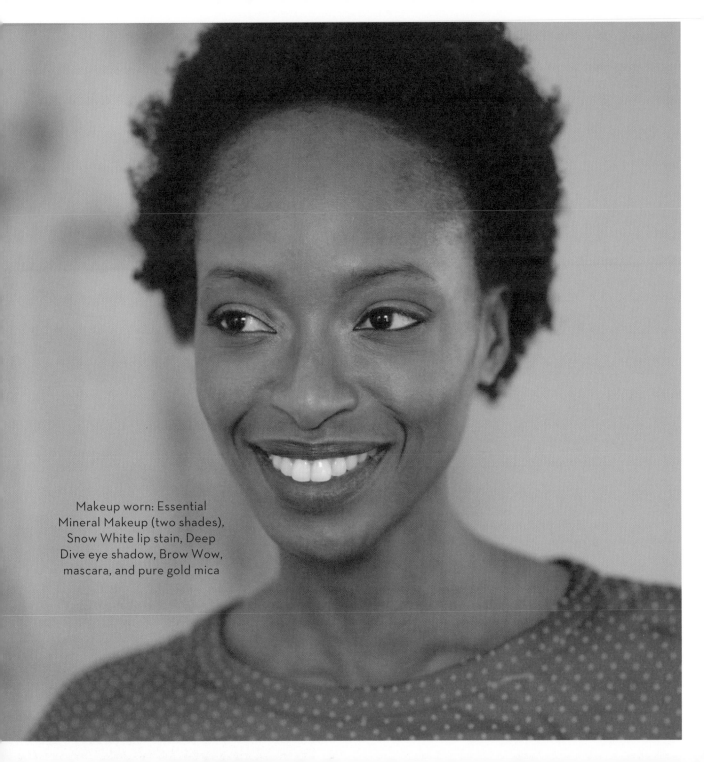

Makeup worn: Essential Mineral Makeup (two shades), Snow White lip stain, Deep Dive eye shadow, Brow Wow, mascara, and pure gold mica

COLOR PALETTE BLENDS

Top Shelf

COGNAC

A deep, rich brown with a hint of bronze shimmer.

2 teaspoons Eye Shadow Powder Base, prepared (page 121)

$1/8$ **teaspoon black iron oxide**

$3/32$ **teaspoon red iron oxide**

$3/32$ **teaspoon yellow iron oxide**

$1/16$ **teaspoon bronze mica**

BRANDY

A cool brown midtone.

2 teaspoons Eye Shadow Powder Base, prepared (page 121)

$1/8$ **teaspoon titanium dioxide**

$3/32$ **teaspoon yellow iron oxide**

$3/32$ **teaspoon brown iron oxide**

Speck of red iron oxide

CHAMPAGNE

A soft, effervescent gold.

2 teaspoons Eye Shadow Powder Base, prepared (page 121)

$1/16$ **teaspoon titanium dioxide**

$1/64$ **teaspoon yellow iron oxide**

$1/128$ **teaspoon brown iron oxide**

$1/32$ **teaspoon gold mica**

Speck red iron oxide

Desert Dunes

DESERT SAND

A cool, dusty beige.

2 teaspoons Eye Shadow Powder Base, prepared (page 121)

$1/16$ **teaspoon titanium dioxide**

$1/32$ **teaspoon yellow iron oxide**

$1/32$ **teaspoon brown iron oxide**

Speck of red iron oxide

DESERT ASH

This pale gray has just a hint of warmth to it.

2 teaspoons Eye Shadow Powder Base, prepared (page 121)

$1/8$ **teaspoon titanium dioxide**

$1/8$ **teaspoon black iron oxide**

$1/8$ **teaspoon brown iron oxide**

DESERT SHADOW

A rich, warm brown with a hint of dust.

2 teaspoons Eye Shadow Powder Base, prepared (page 121)

$1/8$ **teaspoon black iron oxide**

$1/8$ **teaspoon red iron oxide**

$1/8$ **teaspoon yellow iron oxide**

DESERT GREEN

A strong, cool khaki.

2 teaspoons Eye Shadow Powder Base, prepared (page 121)

1/8 teaspoon green chromium oxide

1/8 teaspoon brown iron oxide

Deep Dive

MIDNIGHT BLUE

A deep, dark black-blue with a hint of golden shimmer.

2 teaspoons Eye Shadow Powder Base, prepared (page 121)

1/4 teaspoon black iron oxide

1/8 teaspoon blue ultramarine

1/16 teaspoon gold mica

OPEN OCEAN

This crisp, clear blue is reminiscent of the open ocean on a sunny day.

2 teaspoons Eye Shadow Powder Base, prepared (page 121)

1/4 teaspoon blue ultramarine

1/16 teaspoon black iron oxide

1/16 teaspoon silver mica

TIDE POOL

A rich, cool turquoise with a hint of shimmer.

2 teaspoons Eye Shadow Powder Base, prepared (page 121)

1/4 teaspoon green hydrated chromium oxide

1/32 teaspoon black iron oxide

1/16 teaspoon gold mica

1/32 teaspoon blue ultramarine

PARADISE

Daydream of the beach with this bright turquoise.

2 teaspoons Eye Shadow Powder Base, prepared (page 121)

1/4 teaspoon green hydrated chromium oxide

1/16 teaspoon green chromium oxide

1/16 teaspoon silver mica

1/32 teaspoon blue ultramarine

CREATE YOUR OWN!

When you want to create your own blends there really aren't any hard or fast rules. I've found a ratio of 5/16 teaspoon of pigment to 2 teaspoons base is a good place to start for a fairly strong eye shadow, but you can absolutely use more or less pigment depending on your skin tone and how strong you like your eye shadow.

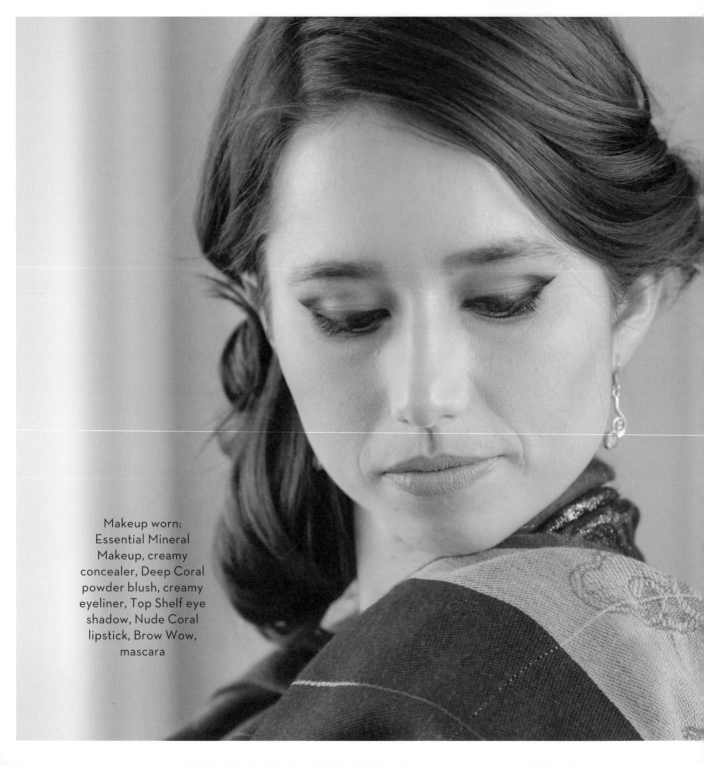

Makeup worn: Essential Mineral Makeup, creamy concealer, Deep Coral powder blush, creamy eyeliner, Top Shelf eye shadow, Nude Coral lipstick, Brow Wow, mascara

Creamy eyeliner

Apparently I expect a lot from my eyeliner. I want to put it on and leave it there, and have it stay where I put it from morning to night (and potentially to the following morning as well). It turns out that this is quite a lot to expect from eyeliner. Many of my shop-bought oil-based eyeliners (aka pencil liners) can't do this, so when it came to developing my own formula, I knew some extensive experimentation was in order.

I quickly accumulated a large collection of carefully numbered wee dishes full of black waxy concoctions that I'd paint onto my face and watch melt off. I'd go into the office for the day with different formulas on each eye and end up with noticeably lopsided wear by lunchtime.

Through my experiments I noticed that softer eyeliners applied beautifully, but smudged off in minutes (sometimes my eyeliner would be a mess before I even left for work). As I increased the amount of wax in the formulas they'd stay on longer, but not that much longer, and the resulting eyeliner was pretty terrible. Those higher wax formulas were skiddy and awful to apply, offering no precision and quite a lot of frustration (imagine trying to use a cheap crayon as eyeliner—ugh!). So, I decided to loop in some of my awesome primers (page 118–119) with a creamier formula and see what happened. That turned out to be a fantastic combination. A creamy eyeliner paired with either of my eye primers gives you eyeliner that can be applied precisely (or smudged to your heart's content) and then stays in place

for hours on end (paired with my Powdered Eye Primer [page 118] I've slept in this eyeliner after a full day of wear and it didn't budge—it basically becomes a long-wearing gel eyeliner). It's the best of both worlds! If you don't want to pair this eyeliner with primer, you'll find the wear is similar to that of a soft kohl eyeliner.

The base of my eyeliner is a blend of jojoba and castor oils that have been thickened with beeswax and candelilla wax. While these ingredients will make a thick, creamy eyeliner when paired with iron oxides, that eyeliner will not stay in place, so we give it a hand with two adhesion-boosting ingredients. Magnesium stearate is fantastic for both slip and adhesion, helping combat the skid that can happen in higher-wax formulations and helping the eyeliner stay in place, while magnesium myristate is a bit of an adhesion miracle in everything (you'll notice it in a lot of my eye makeup formulas).

My favorite thing about this base recipe is how easy it is to whip up a batch and turn it into different colors of eyeliners whenever you want.

You can easily melt up a batch now and keep it on hand, scooping out some of it as needed and transforming it with all kinds of wonderful pigments and micas to make a rainbow of eyeliners (I once made a green and gold eyeliner on Christmas Eve to wear to a party an hour later!). From classic black to bright aquamarine to gold, consider the world of eyeliner yours to conquer.

Each color blend will make approximately 0.17 ounce (5 g) of eyeliner. Compare that to the size of a standard shop-bought cream or gel eyeliner, which is around 0.1 ounce (3 g)!

Creamy Eyeliner Base

MAKES APPROXIMATELY 1.48 OUNCES (42 G)

0.33 ounce (10 g) refined beeswax

0.1 ounce (3 g) candelilla wax

0.45 ounce (13 g) jojoba oil

0.45 ounce (13 g) castor oil

10 drops vitamin E oil

1¼ teaspoon magnesium stearate

Scant teaspoon magnesium myristate

Pigment (see Creamy Eyeliner Color Blends section on page 130)

Using your digital scale, weigh the beeswax, candelilla wax, jojoba oil, and castor oil into a small saucepan. Measure out the magnesium stearate and magnesium myristate and add those to the saucepan as well. Stir everything together with a flexible silicone spatula to break up the powders and thoroughly incorporate them into the oils before melting everything over low, direct heat (as opposed to a water bath). We're melting this base over direct heat because magnesium stearate has a high enough melting point (190°F [88°C]) that melting it in a water bath is quite difficult and time-consuming, especially if you live at higher elevations. Keep a close eye on the base as it melts so it doesn't scorch. If it does scorch, you'll need to throw it out and start over or you'll find your eyeliner has a strange, curdled appearance to it when you've added the pigments, and it won't apply or wear well (it'll also smell odd). As the base melts, you'll reach a point where it's liquid, but appears cloudy—this cloudiness is from unmelted magnesium stearate and magnesium myristate. You're not done melting until those powders have melted, leaving the liquid eyeliner base golden and transparent. Remove the base from the heat as soon as everything has melted; this will take about 30 minutes over low heat. Voilà, you have eyeliner base.

Now it's time to start adding pigment!

Once you have your base you're ready to turn it into a rainbow of colors. Each color will require 0.14 ounce (4 g) of eyeliner base, which you'll want to weigh out into a small glass or metal bowls (aim for 1/2 cup [125 mL] or less in size). You can weigh out the base while it's still liquid or let it set up and measure it as a solid, whichever you prefer is fine, but I find measuring it as a solid is significantly easier.

Because you'll need to remelt the base to incorporate the pigments, prepare a water bath by bringing about 1 inch (2.5 cm) of water to a not-quite simmer (it should just be steaming hot) in a wide, shallow pan. Add the pigments to your small bowl of eyeliner base and place that bowl in your water bath to allow the base to melt, which should take about 5 minutes. Using a flexible silicone spatula, stir and blend everything together. You can leave the bowl in the water bath as you blend the pigments in, or remove it to stir if you're finding the steam too

hot on your hands. Place the bowl back in the water bath to remelt the eyeliner as needed. Smear the spatula against the bottom of the bowl to break up clumps of pigment. When you can no longer see streaks of distinct colors on the bottom of the dish when you drag your spatula across it (this will take 3 to 5 minutes of stirring and blending) and the eyeliner is smooth and uniform in color, you're done!

Pour your finished eyeliner into a 0.17-ounce (5 g) jar and let it solidify before using. It will only take about 30 minutes for your eyeliner to solidify enough to use, but it will continue to harden for up to 24 hours after you pour it, so don't be surprised if it seems too soft at first.

Because this eyeliner is entirely oil-based, we aren't worried about mold. The oils in it will eventually oxidize and go rancid, but the vitamin E will help delay that so you should get at least a year out of these eyeliners before that happens if you store them somewhere cool and dry. If your eyeliner starts to smell like crayons or old nuts, the oils have gone rancid, so chuck it out and make some more.

Tip: I like to apply this eyeliner with a pencil-tipped eyeliner brush, but an angle brush will work as well. You can purchase empty eyeliner pencils, but I've found filling them to be more work (and mess) than it's worth.

CREAMY EYELINER COLOR BLENDS

BLACK

0.14 ounce (4 g) Creamy Eyeliner Base, prepared (page 128)

$7/16$ teaspoon black iron oxide

PLUM PURPLE

0.14 ounce (4 g) Creamy Eyeliner Base, prepared (page 128)

$3/8$ teaspoon blue ultramarine

$1/16$ teaspoon carmine

$1/16$ teaspoon red iron oxide

WARM BROWN SHIMMER

0.14 ounce (4 g) Creamy Eyeliner Base, prepared (page 128)

$5/16$ teaspoon brown iron oxide

$1/16$ teaspoon yellow iron oxide

$1/16$ teaspoon red iron oxide

$1/16$ teaspoon bronze mica

OLIVE

0.14 ounce (4 g) Creamy Eyeliner Base, prepared (page 128)

$1/4$ teaspoon brown iron oxide

$1/16$ teaspoon yellow iron oxide

$1/8$ teaspoon brown iron oxide

$1/16$ teaspoon gold mica

FOREST GREEN

0.14 ounce (4 g) Creamy Eyeliner Base, prepared (page 128)

$5/16$ teaspoon chromium green oxide

$1/8$ teaspoon black iron oxide

BRIGHT TURQUOISE

0.14 ounce (4 g) Creamy Eyeliner Base, prepared (page 128)

$7/16$ teaspoon hydrated chromium oxide

CREATE YOUR OWN!

To blend up your own colors, the rule of thumb is $7/16$ teaspoon of pigment per 4 g of base, with up to $1/16$ teaspoon of mica on top of that.

Tip: I said this in the introduction to this chapter but it bears repeating: because this eyeliner isn't at all waterproof, please don't tightline with it! It'll quickly come off and irritate your eyes.

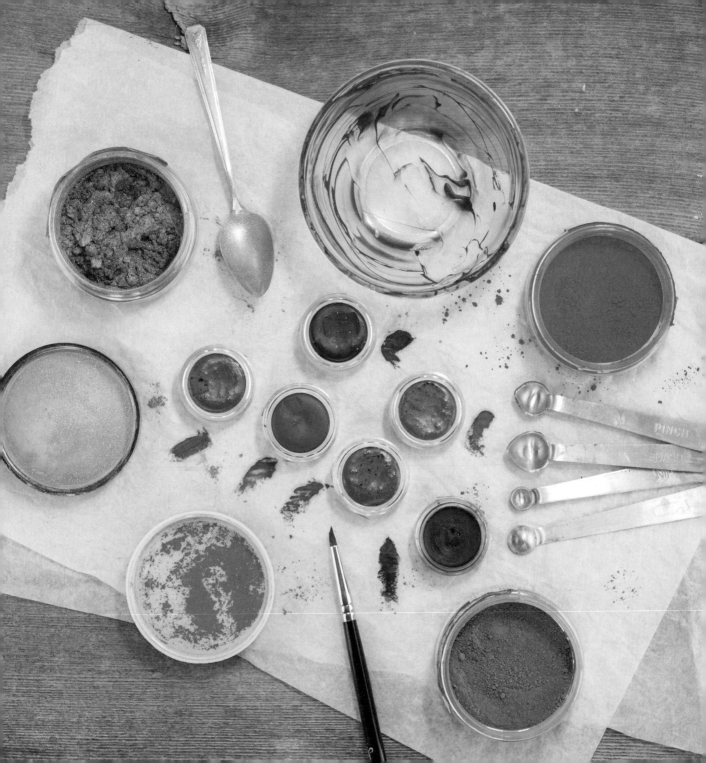

GEL EYELINER

This gel eyeliner is quite the thrill (to me, at least). It's incredibly easy to make (mostly just whisking), beyond easy to customize, and super flexible. It goes on like paint, dries quickly, and stays on beautifully for a solid 10 hours or more! If that's not impressive, I don't know what is. Pair it with my Powdered Eye Primer (page 118) for incredibly long wear.

The base of this gel eyeliner is wonderfully simple—it's xanthan gum and water. Xanthan (pronounced zan-than) gum is a polysaccharide that is a powerful and stable thickener in teensy amounts. It's also what allows our powders and pigments to stay suspended in our base. Whisking a wee bit of xanthan gum into water gives us a thick gel, and from there we'll build our eyeliners by adding colors (in the form of oxides and other powdered pigments) and adhesion helpers, like glycerin, magnesium myristate, and castor oil.

You can use this gel eyeliner two ways. My personal preference is to let it dry out completely, and then use it like watercolor paint—simply wet your brush before use. I love this because you can vary the strength of the liner by using different amounts of water, and it's easier to travel with when leaking isn't a concern. You can definitely leave your eyeliner hydrated, but it's a bit of a battle trying to stop it from drying out, and I find it's harder to apply, so I suppose I just like to embrace the inevitable!

Tip: Be sure to store your xanthan gum somewhere cool and dry, in a well-sealed bag with all the air squeezed out. If it gets damp, it'll be much harder to work with.

Gel Eyeliner Base

MAKES 0.53 OUNCE (15 G)

$^1/_{16}$ teaspoon xanthan gum

1 tablespoon (15 mL) just-boiled water

Broad-spectrum preservative (follow manufacturer's recommendation for usage amount; 1 percent would be approximately 0.0053 ounce [0.15 g])

Pigment (see Gel Eyeliner Color Blends section on page 135)

Prepare a water bath by bringing about 1 inch (2.5 cm) of water to a not-quite simmer (it should just be steaming hot) in a wide, shallow pan.

Measure the just-boiled water out into a small glass or metal bowl (something that holds approximately half a cup [125 mL]) and pop it in the hot water bath. Xanthan gum is very prone to clumping in even slightly cool water, so we'll prevent clumps by keeping our wee dish of water hot as we work.

Slowly sprinkle small amounts of xanthan gum over the water in the dish, whisking vigorously between additions with a tiny wire whisk. You should notice the water start to thicken quite quickly, and little air bubbles will form as you whisk away. Once you've added all the xanthan gum, you should have a thick blob of water that slides around in its dish a bit when tilted. Whisk in your preservative, and now it's time to turn that base into eyeliner!

You'll need to make your eyeliner directly after making the gel base as it dries out quite quickly. Fortunately the base is simple and inexpensive to make, so no worries if you need to toss some of it out and make more later. You'll turn this base into eyeliner in the following steps.

Now it's time to start adding pigment!

To turn the base into eyeliner, start by choosing a color blend recipe. Weigh 0.03 ounce (1g) of the gel base out into a small bowl (think $^1/_3$ cup [80 mL] or smaller) and top with the remaining ingredients for the color blend. Whisk thoroughly with your miniature wire whisk until all the powders are completely incorporated (this will take about 1 minute) and you are left with a thick, highly pigmented gel. You just made eyeliner! Use a thin silicone spatula to scrape it up and transfer it to a small container (0.17 ounce [5 g] or 0.1 ounce [3 g]) and leave it uncapped to dry out (this will take 2 or 3 days; you'll know it's dry when it feels quite solid and is no longer shiny in appearance). Use it like watercolor paint once it's dried by getting your brush wet and working up some eyeliner to apply.

Because this gel eyeliner contains water (and will continue to come into contact with water even if you let it dry out), it is susceptible to mold growth and microbial spoilage, which is why we've included a broad-spectrum preservative. Preservatives are especially important to include for things that contain water that we're putting around our eyes—do not leave it out! If you notice any changes in the scent, texture, or mold population department, throw it away and make more.

Tip: Some pigments are better in gel eyeliners than others; you'll find the ultramarines are difficult to incorporate into the gel base and can seem to separate a bit in the container (though the color is still uniform when you go to apply it).

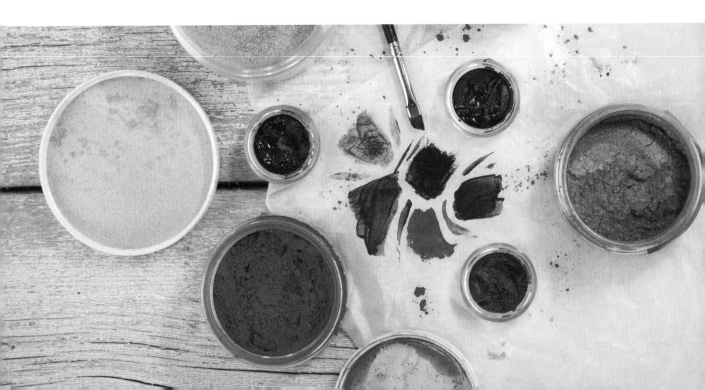

GEL EYELINER COLOR BLENDS

Classic Black Gel Eyeliner

MAKES APPROXIMATELY 0.07 OUNCE (2 G)

0.03 ounce (1 g) Gel Eyeliner Base, prepared (page 133)
1/4 teaspoon black iron oxide
1/64 teaspoon magnesium myristate
4 drops castor oil
7 drops vegetable glycerin

Eggplant Purple Gel Eyeliner

MAKES APPROXIMATELY 0.07 OUNCE (2 G)

0.03 ounce (1 g) Gel Eyeliner Base, prepared (page 133)
3/16 teaspoon blue ultramarine
1/16 teaspoon carmine
1/64 teaspoon magnesium myristate
4 drops castor oil
7 drops vegetable glycerin

Midnight Ocean Gel Eyeliner

MAKES APPROXIMATELY 0.07 OUNCE (2 G)

0.03 ounce (1 g) Gel Eyeliner Base, prepared (page 133)
3/16 teaspoon blue ultramarine
1/16 teaspoon black iron oxide
1/64 teaspoon magnesium myristate
4 drops castor oil
7 drops vegetable glycerin

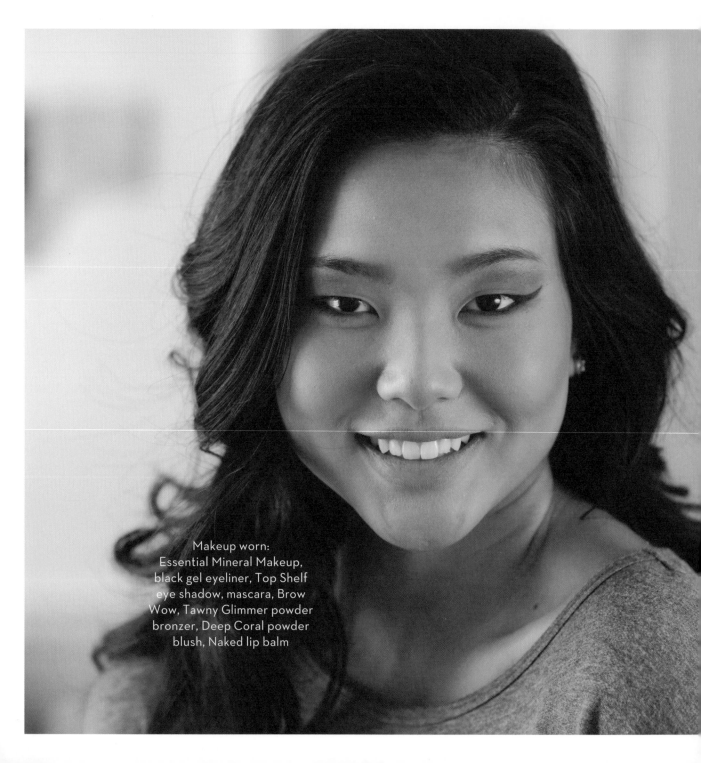

Makeup worn:
Essential Mineral Makeup,
black gel eyeliner, Top Shelf
eye shadow, mascara, Brow
Wow, Tawny Glimmer powder
bronzer, Deep Coral powder
blush, Naked lip balm

Coffee Gel Eyeliner

MAKES APPROXIMATELY 0.07 OUNCE (2 G)

0.03 ounce (1 g) Gel Eyeliner Base, prepared (page 133)

$^1/_4$ teaspoon brown iron oxide

$^1/_{64}$ teaspoon magnesium myristate

4 drops castor oil

7 drops vegetable glycerin

Electric Turquoise Gel Eyeliner

MAKES APPROXIMATELY 0.07 OUNCE (2G)

0.03 ounce (1 g) Gel Eyeliner Base, prepared (page 133)

$^1/_4$ teaspoon green hydrated chromium oxide

$^1/_{64}$ teaspoon magnesium myristate

4 drops castor oil

7 drops vegetable glycerin

·········· CREATE YOUR OWN! ··········

General rule for creating your own eyeliner color blend: 1 g base, $^1/_4$ teaspoon pigment, up to $^1/_{16}$ teaspoon mica (optional), $^1/_{64}$ teaspoon magnesium myristate, 4 drops castor oil, and 7 drops vegetable glycerin. Have fun!

Tip: This eyeliner isn't at all waterproof, so please don't tightline with it! It will come off quickly and irritate your eyes.

Mascara

HOMEMADE MASCARA IS HARD. MASCARA OCCUPIES A COSMETIC PARADOX. IT MUST DRY QUICKLY ONCE on your eyelashes, but not on the brush or in the container. It mustn't dry so much that it flakes, nor so little that it melts off. It needs to stay on all day, and then come off with relative ease when you're through with it. All that is to say that devising a formula for homemade mascara is quite challenging. I've tossed so many wee pots of black goo over the years that I was starting to think I would never find something that worked, and then one day I noticed how a clay mask coats any stray hairs it comes into contact with, and I had a brainwave.

This mascara formula is a few generations past my first successful formula. I've tweaked it so we don't need to get our pigment from the clay, resulting in a far more accessible (and inexpensive) ingredient list.

I'd recommend keeping the final product in a small (around 0.49 ounce [14 g]) sealing jar that's wide and reasonably shallow. That will allow you to run a mascara brush across the top of it without losing the last of your mascara. You can purchase empty mascara tubes, but I've never been that taken with them—they're a pain to fill. I'd also advise against trying to clean out an old mascara tube and reuse it; it is an exercise in futility. Old mascara tubes contain a never-ending black hole of black tarry paste, and even if you ever did manage to flush it all out, the hole at the top of the tube is too narrow to refill it. I learned the hard way so you don't have to!

I've kept this mascara fairly dry, leaving you to dampen your mascara brush a bit before you apply it. This allows you to vary how thick you want your mascara to be each time you apply it. More water makes for more of a lash tint, while less water gives you a lengthening, thickening mascara (be sure to scrape any excess mascara off your brush on the edge of the jar before applying it to prevent clumpy lashes). You can also experiment with the brush you use for different effects! Mascara brushes from purchased tubes are something you can clean and save, soaking them in liberal amounts of high-proof rubbing alcohol to get them clean before using. I love being able to use those crazy spiky wands with my homemade mascara! Pair with curled lashes for the best effect.

0.07 ounce (2 g) refined beeswax

0.03 ounce (1 g) Emulsifying
Wax NF, BTMS-50, or Polawax

0.03 ounce (1 g) jojoba oil

0.03 ounce (1 g) vegetable glycerin

0.21 ounce (6 g) water

$^1/_2$ teaspoon white kaolin clay

1 teaspoon black iron oxide

Broad-spectrum preservative
(follow manufacturer's
recommendation for usage
amount; 1 percent is approximately 0.0049 ounce [0.14 g])

Prepare a water bath by bringing about 1 inch (2.5 cm) of water to a not-quite simmer (it should just be steaming hot) in a wide, shallow pan.

Measure all the ingredients, minus the preservative, into a small glass or metal bowl (aim for one that holds approximately $^1/_2$ cup [125 mL]) and place that bowl in the water bath to melt everything through, which will take about 10 minutes. Once everything has melted, remove the bowl from the heat, dry off the outside, and use a miniature wire whisk to blend in the preservative.

Keep whisking the mascara as it cools. Depending on which emulsifying wax you used, one of two things will happen. If you used Polawax or Emulsifying Wax NF, as everything emulsifies you'll find you have a somewhat thick creamy black lotion that's definitely liquid. After you blend in your preservative, pour the mascara into a 0.33 ounce (10 g) container with a sealing lid; over the next few days the mascara will thicken up to more of a semi-solid paste.

If you used BTMS-50 as your emulsifying wax, your mascara will thicken up to a stiff paste within a few minutes of whisking, so be sure you add your preservative within a minute of removing your mascara from the heat or you'll find it quite difficult to evenly incorporate. Scrape your mascara into a 0.33 ounce (10 g) container with a sealing lid, and at this point it's as thick as it'll get.

To apply, wet a mascara brush with a drop or two of water and run your brush across the surface of your mascara, scraping any excess off on the edge of the jar before applying as usual. And avoid getting the mascara in your eyes and on your waterline!

Because this mascara contains water, it is susceptible to

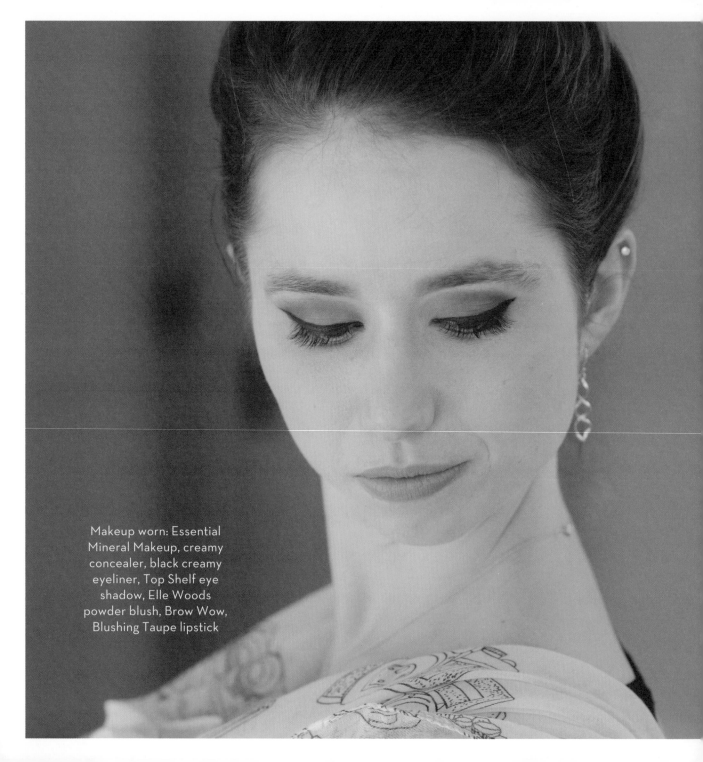

Makeup worn: Essential
Mineral Makeup, creamy
concealer, black creamy
eyeliner, Top Shelf eye
shadow, Elle Woods
powder blush, Brow Wow,
Blushing Taupe lipstick

mold growth and microbial spoilage, which is why we've included a broad-spectrum preservative. Preservatives are especially important to include for things that contain water that we're putting around our eyes—do not leave it out! If you notice any changes in the scent, texture, or mold population department, chuck it and make more.

Tip: While there are lots of emulsifying waxes available, I've found the three I've suggested don't irritate my eyes. In most applications that call for a complete emulsifying wax, one variety is generally easily swapped for another without any impact on the final product, but I've found that other emulsifying waxes I tried made my eyes burn, so I'd recommend sticking with Polawax (cetearyl alcohol, PEG-150 Stearate, Polysorbate 60, and Steareth-20), BTMS-50 (behentrimonium methosulfate, cetyl alcohol, and butylene glycol), or Emulsifying Wax NF (cetostearyl alcohol and Polysorbate 60).

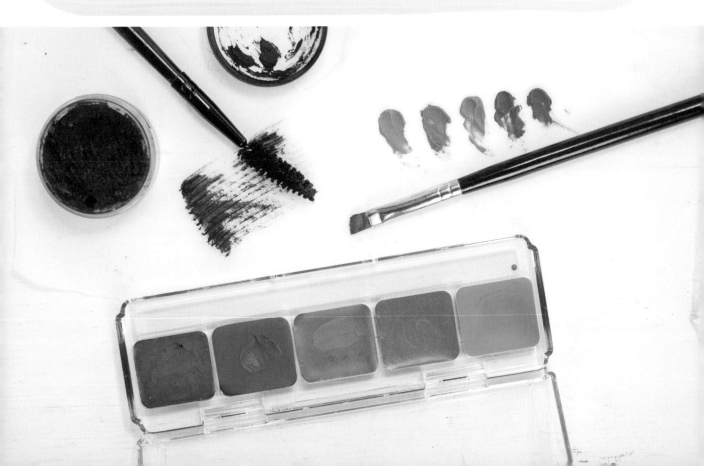

Brow Wow

I'D BE THE FIRST PERSON TO ADMIT THAT I ARRIVED AT THE BROW PARTY PRETTY LATE, AND IN A FAIRLY ODD way. I was at the Glasgow International Airport painfully early to catch my flight back to Canada, and with plenty of time before boarding, I agreed to a 5 a.m. makeover at the duty-free shop. The lovely makeup artist chatted to me in her fantastic Scottish accent as she filled in my brows, erased my pores, and did all sorts of other cosmetic magic. When she was done I liked what I saw. Filled-in brows frame and highlight my eyes in a subtle, natural-looking way. I've been a convert ever since.

This brow fixative is a thick, oil-based cream that coats and darkens the hairs, as well as settling them in place. You can pair it with matching powder (just use some homemade eye shadow—page 121) to set everything and fill in any gaps if you need to. The creamy part should be roughly the same color as your brows, while the powder should be lighter than the cream by a few shades. I've developed five blends for different complexions to get you started.

MAKES APPROXIMATELY
0.25 OUNCE (7 G)

0.1 ounce (3 g) refined beeswax
0.14 ounce (4 g) jojoba oil
4 drops vitamin E oil
$^1/_8$ teaspoon magnesium stearate
$^1/_{32}$ teaspoon titanium dioxide
$^1/_{32}$ teaspoon sericite mica
$^1/_8$ teaspoon calcium carbonate
FAIR
$^1/_{32}$ teaspoon titanium dioxide
$^1/_{32}$ teaspoon brown iron oxide
LIGHT
$^1/_{32}$ teaspoon brown iron oxide

Weigh the beeswax, jojoba oil, vitamin E, and magnesium stearate out into a small saucepan and blend together with a flexible silicone spatula, taking care to break up any clumps of magnesium stearate and blend them into the oils to help everything melt faster. Place the saucepan on the burner over low heat and melt through, stirring to ensure everything melts evenly (this will take about 10 minutes). We're melting this over direct heat instead of in a water bath because of the relatively high melting point of magnesium stearate; it doesn't melt well in water baths. Take care not to scorch the mixture, removing it from the heat as soon as everything has melted and the mixture is transparent (un-melted magnesium stearate will make the otherwise melted base appear cloudy).

As the oil mixture melts, measure your pigments, the titanium dioxide, the sericite mica, and the calcium carbonate

MEDIUM

$^1/_{32}$ teaspoon brown iron oxide,

$^1/_{32}$ black iron oxide

DARK

$^1/_{64}$ teaspoon brown iron oxide

$^3/_{64}$ teaspoon black iron oxide

DARKEST

$^3/_{64}$ teaspoon brown iron oxide

$^1/_{8}$ teaspoon + $^1/_{64}$ teaspoon
   black iron oxide

out into a small glass or metal bowl ($^1/_2$ cup [125 mL] or less). Once your oils have melted, pour them into the bowl with the powders and blend everything together with a flexible silicone spatula. You will need to pop the bowl into a shallow pan of not-quite simmering water to re-melt the base as it'll likely solidify before you're done blending in the powders.

Use the spatula to blend in the pigments, smearing the spatula against the sides and bottom of the bowl to break up any clumps of pigment—you'll see distinct streaks of color across the bottom of the bowl as you draw your spatula across it, breaking down the pigments. Once you have a smooth, evenly colored mixture, pour it into a 0.35-ounce (10 g) container and let it set up for at least 2 hours before using. It will only take about 10 minutes for your Brow Wow to appear solid, but it will still be too soft to use. I like to use an angled eyeliner brush to comb Brow Wow through my eyebrows, using fairly little product and building up to the look I want.

Because this brow wax is entirely oil-based we aren't worried about mold, but the oils will eventually oxidize and go rancid. Thanks to the vitamin E in the recipe you should get at least a year out of your Brow Wow if you store it in a relatively cool and dry place. If your Brow Wow starts to smell like crayons or old nuts, that's a sign that the oils have oxidized and it's time to make a new batch.

Tip: The calcium carbonate in this recipe helps keeps your brows from looking greasy.

CHAPTER SIX:

LIP MAKEUP

Welcome to the never-ending rainbow of homemade lip color. With recipes for everything from lip gloss to lipstick to lip stain, you'll never find yourself wishing for the perfect shade again. From classic reds to bright corals to vibrant purples, prepare to pucker up!

TINTED LIP BALM

Tinted lip balms are crazy simple: take lip balm, add color. You're done. That's it. We'll mostly be using micas and oxides for the color part. Micas are mesmerizingly shimmery and available in a rainbow of beautiful colors, but they aren't very potent. They'll color the lip balm, but not your lips unless you use quite a lot (though they'll definitely bring the shimmer party!). Potent iron oxides add color in a variety of earthy colors. We'll look at recipes that use both, and a combination of the two (and a few other options, too).

Both iron oxides and micas are fine insoluble powders. Because the powders are insoluble, the small particle size is important—it means we won't feel bits of gritty pigment in the lip balm when it's done; that would be seriously unpleasant. Since the lip balm base is entirely oil-based, oil-soluble dyes are also a good choice for making tinted lip balms. You can purchase many of the iron oxides pre-dispersed in oils for an easier-to-incorporate option, and there are some plant-derived oil-soluble dyes as well.

Carmine is also fantastic in tinted lip balms for a beautiful, cool pink shade. The powder version incorporates nicely with a bit of stirring, and there's also an oil-soluble liquid dye that is often much less expensive than the powdered version and works really well (though it's obviously not suited for powdered cosmetics like blush).

There are also some lovely water-soluble tinting options out there, like alkanet root and madder root. Both are the roots of different plants, and are often available as powders. Because these powders are water-soluble, we can't add them straight to the oils or we'll end up with a nicely colored lip scrub (eek). We can, however, infuse their color into the oils, like making a cup of tea. Some herbs infuse better than others, and since we are dealing with plants, colors can vary between batches and suppliers. Herbs aren't as reliable as oxides and micas, but there's something to be said for the loveliness of an herb-infused balm. We'll make one of those, too.

We already made some Naked Lip Balm (page 49) with beeswax back in the starter projects section, so here we'll add a vegan alternative to that lip balm for anybody who wants to avoid animal products, or for people who like a glossier lip balm. We're using plant-based candelilla wax to thicken this lip balm instead of beeswax. Candelilla is hard and glassy, meaning we need less of it to thicken up the oils and end up with a balmy final product. Beyond the wax change, though, these two bases are basically the same, making them easily interchangeable. Choose your base, choose your color, and we're ready to roll!

Vegan Lip Balm Base

MAKES ELEVEN 0.15 OUNCE (4.25 G) TUBES OF LIP BALM

0.28 ounce (8 g) candelilla wax

0.42 ounce (12 g) virgin coconut oil

0.28 ounce (8 g) cocoa butter

0.67 ounce (19 g) sweet almond oil or safflower oil

6 drops vitamin E oil

20 drops essential oil (optional—I like peppermint)

Pigment (see Lip Balm Color Blends section on page 148)

Beeswax Lip Balm Base

MAKES ELEVEN 0.15 OUNCE (4.25 G) TUBES OF LIP BALM

0.35 ounce (10 g) beeswax

0.42 ounce (12 g) virgin coconut oil

0.25 ounce (7 g) cocoa butter

0.67 ounce (19 g) sweet almond oil or safflower oil

6 drops vitamin E oil

20 drops essential oil (optional—I like peppermint)

Pigment (see Lip Balm Color Blends section on page 148)

PREPARE A WATER BATH BY BRINGING ABOUT 2 INCHES (5 CM) OF WATER TO A GENTLE SIMMER IN A SMALL saucepan. Up next, choose your base. Weigh the ingredients (except the essential oils) into a heat-resistant glass measuring cup—choose one with a pouring spout for easier pouring at the end.

Place the measuring cup of ingredients into your water bath to melt everything together.

Let the oils melt in the water bath for at least 25 minutes before removing the measuring cup from the heat. The oils will melt well before 25 minutes pass, but this extra time thoroughly heats the measuring cup up as well, giving us more time to stir in the pigments before the oils start to cool and thicken. While the oils melt, set out twelve 0.15 ounce (4.25 g) lip balm tubes (I find lining them up so they're touching helps minimize spills). Dry the measuring cup off after removing it from the water bath to prevent accidentally getting water in the lip balm. You'll finish off the lip balm by adding tinting ingredients, in the following steps.

Now it's time to start adding pigment!

Measure your selected pigments into the measuring cup of melted oils and thoroughly blend the pigments into the lip balm base with a flexible silicone spatula, taking care to break up any powdery clumps by smearing the spatula against the bottom and sides of the measuring cup—this will take 2 or 3 minutes. If the base starts to thicken before you're done blending in the pigment, simply place the measuring cup back in the water bath for a minute or so to remelt it.

Once the liquid lip balm has cooled enough to be the consistency of coffee creamer and is uniformly colored, with no noticeable clumps of pigment, it's time to pour it into the lip balm tubes (if you're adding any essential oils, stir them in directly before pouring). As you get down toward the bottom of the liquid lip balm you might notice there's some visible, sand-like bits of pigment leftover. Leave those in the bottom of the measuring cup rather than scraping them out into the last lip balm tube or that last lip balm will be unpleasantly gritty.

Now all that's left is to let your lip balm set up and you're all done! This will take about 10 minutes, and you'll know they've set because the color will lighten a bit and the lip balm will be opaque and uniform. Once they've set up, label them so you'll remember what they are.

Because this tinted lip balm is entirely oil-based, it doesn't require any preservatives to ward off bacterial growth, and the vitamin E in the recipe will help delay the oils going rancid. These lip balms should last at least a year, if not several. Store unopened tubes in the fridge for the longest possible shelf life. If you notice your tube of lip balm has started to smell off, like crayons or old nuts, it's time to toss it and start a new one.

LIP BALM COLOR BLENDS

Sun-Kissed

MICAS BRING A LOVELY BIT OF SHIMMER AND GLIMMER TO A TINTED LIP BALM, AND WHILE THEY'LL ADD some color while the balm is in the tube, they don't contribute much to the lips, meaning this lip balm imparts a seductively subtle sun kiss. You can use gold, copper, or bronze mica—whatever you have on hand or prefer is perfect.

MAKES ELEVEN 0.15 OUNCE (4.25 G) TUBES OF LIP BALM

1 recipe lip balm base, beeswax or vegan, prepared (page 146)

$\frac{1}{4}$ teaspoon gold, bronze, or copper mica

Berry Sorbet

IRON OXIDES ARE POTENT PIGMENTS, MEANING JUST A WEE BIT WILL GIVE US A BEAUTIFULLY TINTED LIP balm. This berry tinted lip balm gets its color from red iron oxide, and its chilly shimmer from a touch of silver mica.

MAKES ELEVEN 0.15 OUNCE (4.25 G) TUBES OF LIP BALM

1 recipe lip balm base, beeswax or vegan, prepared (page 146)

$\frac{1}{8}$ teaspoon red iron oxide • $\frac{1}{8}$ teaspoon silver mica

Popping Pink

THE SMALLEST AMOUNT OF POTENT PINK POWDERED CARMINE TRANSFORMS OUR LIP BALM BASE INTO THE prettiest pink lip tint. You can double the carmine for a stronger color if you love your pink!

MAKES ELEVEN 0.15 OUNCE (4.25 G) TUBES OF LIP BALM

1 recipe lip balm base, beeswax or vegan, prepared (page 146)

$\frac{1}{64}$ teaspoon carmine

Alkanet-Infused Tinted Lip Balm

THIS TINTED LIP BALM GETS ITS PRETTY RUBY HUE FROM ALKANET ROOT, *BATSCHIA CANESCENS*. NATIVE TO the Mediterranean, it produces bright blue flowers and dark red roots that have been used as a dye for hundreds of years. Because alkanet root won't dissolve in oil we'll be infusing the powder into the oils and discarding it (like making tea) instead of adding it directly to the oils, so this one is a bit more involved than the lip balms tinted with mica or oxide.

For added scent, you can add some essential oils (peppermint or lavender are nice choices). If you'd like to dress up your lip balm even more, a bit of shimmery mica (I find both silver and gold pair beautifully with the alkanet color) is also a great addition.

MAKES ELEVEN 0.15 OUNCE
(4.25 G) TUBES OF LIP BALM

- 1 recipe lip balm base, vegan or beeswax, unprepared (page 146)
- 1 teaspoon dried alkanet root powder
- 20 drops essential oil (optional)
- $1/4$ teaspoon gold or silver mica (optional)

Prepare a water bath by bringing about 2 inches (5 cm) of water to a gentle simmer in a small saucepan.

Measure the alkanet root out into an empty disposable paper tea bag and tie it off.

Measure the coconut oil, sweet almond oil, and cocoa butter out into a heat-resistant 1 cup (250 mL) measuring cup—we're leaving the wax out during the infusion, but we'll add it in later. Add an extra 0.1 ounce (3 g) of sweet almond oil to make up for what we'll lose to the tea bag, which will inevitably soak up some oil, and place the tea bag of alkanet root powder in the oils.

Put the measuring cup of oils and alkanet root in the hot water bath to melt the oils and butters together (this should take about 5 minutes) before lowering the heat to keep the water warm and allow the alkanet root to infuse in the oils for an hour, taking care not to let the saucepan simmer dry. You can infuse the oils for longer if that's where your day takes you, but I find an hour is plenty of time. Feel free to turn the stove off and let most of the infusing happen at room temperature if you're going to be steeping for longer than an hour so that you don't have to fuss with keeping the pot from simmering dry.

Once your oil mixture has steeped for at least an hour, remove the tea bag of alkanet root, gently pressing it with the back of a spoon to squeeze out as much infused oil as possible, taking care not to tear the tea bag. Discard the tea bag.

Weigh the wax into the melted, infused oils, and place the measuring cup back into the water bath. Bring the water bath to a simmer to melt the wax, stirring to combine. While the wax melts, arrange twelve 0.15 ounce (4.25 g) empty lip balm tubes on your countertop, butting them right up against each other to help reduce spills.

Once the wax has melted (this will take about 10 minutes), remove the measuring cup from the water bath and dry it off. If you'd like to any essential oils or mica, now's the time to stir them in.

Pour the liquid lip balm into your pre-arranged lip balm tubes and let them solidify before capping and labeling. This will take about 10 minutes—you'll know they've set up when the tops have contracted a little bit and the lip balm is opaque and uniform. Once they've solidified, cap them and label them.

Because this lip balm is entirely oil-based, it doesn't require any preservatives to ward off bacterial growth, and the vitamin E in the recipe will help delay the oils going rancid. These lip balms should last at least a year, if not several. Store unopened tubes in the fridge for the longest possible shelf life. If you notice your tube of lip balm has started to smell off, like crayons or old nuts, it's time to toss it out and start a new one.

·· **INVENT YOUR OWN!** ··

If you want to step outside the realm of oxides and micas, there's an amazing array of FD&C lake pigments available as oil-soluble liquid dyes and powdered pigments that work beautifully in tinted lip balms and lipsticks. D&C Red Lake No. 7 is a stunning red that looks just like carmine (only significantly cheaper), and is found in many classic red shades.

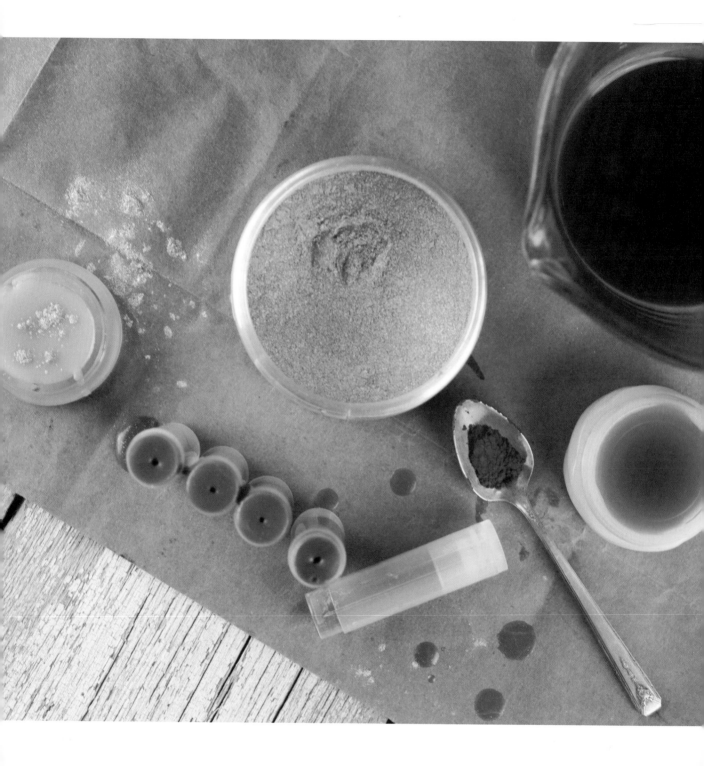

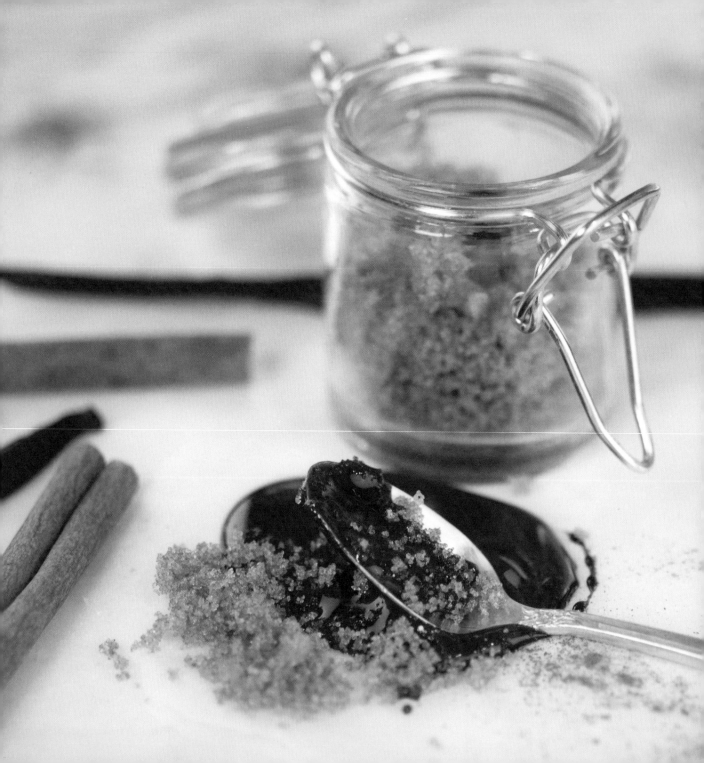

Gingerbread Lip Scrub

THIS SIMPLE SCRUB COMES TOGETHER IN MERE MINUTES, USING INGREDIENTS YOU PROBABLY ALREADY have kicking around your kitchen. Score!

A base of moisturizing coconut oil is combined with classic gingerbread ingredients—sticky molasses, fragrant (and scrubby) ground cinnamon, and exfoliating brown sugar. The resulting scrub tastes fantastic and leaves your lips smooth and hydrated . . . and potentially leaves you craving gingerbread as well!

**MAKES APPROXIMATELY
1 TABLESPOON (15 ML)**

1 teaspoon (5 mL) coconut oil

3 drops vitamin E oil

$1/4$ teaspoon molasses
(blackstrap or fancy)

5 drops vanilla extract

$1/8$ teaspoon ground cinnamon

$1^1/2$ teaspoons brown sugar,
more as needed

Measure the coconut oil and vitamin E out into a small heat-resistant container with a sealing lid—I'd recommend a 4-ounce (118 mL) mason jar. Melt the coconut oil and vitamin E together in the microwave (this will only take about 10 seconds), and then whisk in the molasses and vanilla. Stir in the spices, and then the brown sugar. Add enough brown sugar to mostly absorb the moisture; the scrub should clump up and ooze a little liquid oil.

To use, take about half a teaspoon of the mixture on your fingertip and rub it into your lips over the sink. Rinse off the residue with some water, and enjoy the smoothness!

Tip: Extra lip scrub can be stored in a sealed jar in the fridge for up to 2 weeks. Once the scrub has been chilled the coconut oil will solidify, so you'll find it's much easier to use if you scoop out a useable amount and gently warm it up before use.

Peppermint Sugar Lip Scrub in a Tube

THIS MINTY SCRUB IS BASICALLY JUST LIP BALM WITH ADDED SUGAR. SO IF YOU'VE MADE THE LIP BALM recipe in the starter recipe section (page 146), this scrub will be a cinch. It's all the goodness of lip balm, with added exfoliating goodness. *Parfait!*

The sugar we're using as an exfoliant adds an extra bit of trickiness to the pouring process—the mixture gets to be pretty challenging to pour into lip balm tubes as it cools. It needs to be cool enough that the sugar doesn't settle out of the melted oils, but not so cool that it solidifies and doesn't pour. I find it's best to let the mixture cool most of the way, stirring as it does, before starting to pour. You'll need to work quickly and reheat the mixture in the water bath a few times to keep it at the ideal consistency, but it'll work out in the end.

The final product is a lovely tube of sweet, scrubby, pepperminty delight. After applying the scrub from the tube, use a clean finger (preferably yours) to give your lips a good, firm scrub, and then rinse or wipe off the sugar. The remaining lip balm leaves your lips buffed and moisturized.

MAKES APPROXIMATELY EIGHT 0.15 OUNCE (4.25 G) LIP BALM TUBES

- 0.18 ounce (5 g) beeswax
- 0.21 ounce (6 g) coconut oil
- 0.1 ounce (3 g) cocoa butter
- 0.35 ounce (10 g) sweet almond oil or safflower oil
- 0.03 ounce (1 g) vitamin E oil
- 2 tablespoon granulated white sugar
- 6 drops peppermint essential oil (optional)

Before you get started, prepare your lip balm tubes by lining them up right next to one another on a surface that can be spilled on. I find it's best to have the tubes touching one another as it means you're more likely to spill into another tube than on your countertop! You'll also need to prepare a hot water bath by bringing approximately 2 inches (5 cm) of water to a bare simmer in a small saucepan.

Weigh the beeswax, coconut oil, cocoa butter, sweet almond oil, and vitamin E oil out into a heat-resistant glass measuring cup, and place that measuring cup into your hot water bath. Allow everything to melt (this will take about 10 minutes), and then remove the measuring cup from the water bath. Dry the outside of the measuring cup to avoid getting water in your lip scrub.

Using a flexible spatula, stir in the sugar and essential oil (if using). Stir the mixture as it cools, scooping the sugar up from the bottom as you go. Once you've reached a consistency where the sugar isn't settling out, but the mixture is still pourable, quickly fill your lip balm tubes, reheating and stirring the lip scrub as needed to continue pouring. If the lip scrub is having trouble setting down in the tubes, give them a sharp rap or two on your counter before the scrub solidifies to knock out any air bubbles and force the scrub down the tube.

Because these tubes of lip scrub are entirely oil-based, no broad-spectrum preservatives are required. They should last for at least one year before oxidizing and going rancid. Once you've started using one the scrub is fine to store at room temperature, but I'd recommend storing unused tubes in the fridge for the longest possible shelf life. If you notice your tube of lip scrub starts to smell like crayons or old nuts, it's time to toss it out and start a new one.

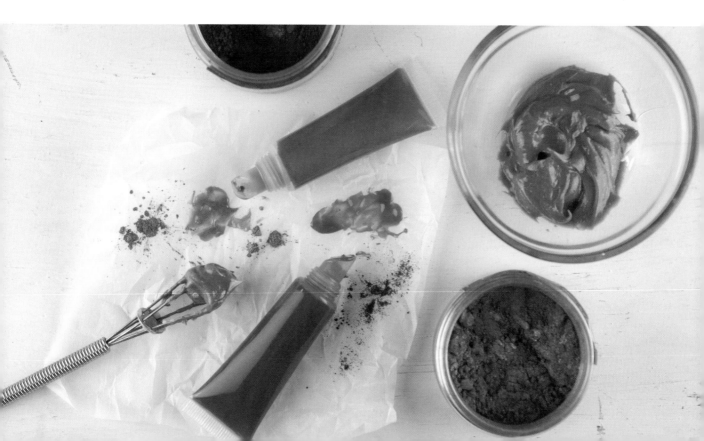

LIP GLOSS

LIP GLOSS IS DELIGHTFULLY SIMPLE. WE'LL ESSENTIALLY MAKE A LIP BALM WITH LESS WAX AND NO BRITTLE cocoa butter, add some shiny castor oil, and then beat in some vegetable glycerin at the end to get a final product that's viscous and shiny. This gives us a base to make any color of lip gloss you can imagine!

You can store your lip gloss in a pot, a hard tube with a wand, or a squeeze tube. Pots are easier to fill, while wands and squeeze tubes are much better for on-the-go applications. If you decide to go either of the tube routes, you'll want to make sure you have a funnel with a tip that will fit in your tube, or a syringe, to make filling possible. Either method will require a good amount of rapping the tube on your counter to knock the lip gloss down the tube to make room for more (be sure to leave room for the wand).

Beeswax Lip Gloss Base

MAKES 1.45 OUNCES (41 G)

0.17 ounce (5 g) beeswax

0.21 ounce (6 g) coconut oil

0.56 ounce (16 g) castor oil

0.35 ounce (10 g) jojoba oil

10 drops vitamin E oil

0.14 ounce (4 g) vegetable glycerin

Broad-spectrum preservative (follow manufacturer's recommendation for usage amount; 1 percent is approximately 0.014 ounce [0.41 g])

Pigment (see Lip Gloss Color Blends section on page 158)

Vegan Lip Gloss Base

MAKES 1.41 OUNCES (40 G)

0.14 ounce (4 g) candelilla wax

0.21 ounce (6 g) coconut oil

0.56 ounce (16 g) castor oil

0.35 ounce (10 g) jojoba oil

10 drops vitamin E oil

0.14 ounce (4 g) vegetable glycerin

Broad-spectrum preservative (follow manufacturer's recommendation for usage amount; 1 percent is approximately 0.014 ounce [0.41 g])

Pigment (see Lip Gloss Color Blends section on page 158)

Prepare a hot water bath by bringing 2 inches (5 cm) of water to a gentle simmer in a small saucepan.

Weigh out the oils and wax into a heat-resistant glass measuring cup. Place the measuring cup in your hot water bath for approximately 10 minutes to melt everything through.

Once all the ingredients have melted, remove the measuring cup from the water bath and dry the outside of it to reduce the chances of accidentally incorporating water into your lip gloss. Stir the melted oils with a flexible spatula periodically as they cool and thicken. While the oils cool, take a few minutes to prepare your containers for filling.

When the oils have cooled to room temperature (this will take about 20 minutes—they'll be opaque and the container will not feel warm to the touch), add the vegetable glycerin and whisk the mixture vigorously until the glycerin emulsifies into the oils, turning into a smooth, uniform lip gloss. This will happen quickly and easily, but the oils *must* be at room temperature.

Because the vegetable glycerin is water-soluble, we will need a broad-spectrum preservative— whisk that in now. If the suggested usage rate is 1 percent, you will need to add approximately 0.014 ounce (0.41 g) of preservative, but be sure to check the recommended usage rate for the specific preservative you are using.

Now it's time to start adding pigment!

The color blends provided here use an entire recipe of this base, but you can easily divide the base up and make a few different kinds of lip gloss from one batch of base. You can also leave the base as it is for a clear lip gloss. To add the pigments, simply whisk them in until the lip gloss is uniform in color; they'll incorporate quite easily, so this will only take about a minute. If you're using essential oils, this is the time to blend them in as well.

After you've blended in your pigments it's time to fill your containers. Because lip gloss is too thick to pour you'll find a syringe or funnel comes in handy to get your gloss into tubes, but you'll be able to spoon it into pots fairly easily.

You should get at least a year of shelf life out of your lip glosses before they spoil. If you notice any changes to the scent, texture, or consistency of your lip gloss it's time to throw it away and make a fresh batch.

LIP GLOSS COLOR BLENDS

Snow White Lip Gloss

THIS PERFECTLY PINK LIP GLOSS GETS ITS FANTASTIC COLOR FROM CARMINE. CARMINE IS MADE FROM the cochineal beetle, so it's natural, but not vegan. Its vibrant, potent color is unmatched elsewhere in nature, though D&C Red Lake No. 7 is a great synthetic alternative. Because Red Lake No. 7 is insoluble it's not always a good alternative for carmine, but it can be used here.

Since carmine is so potent, we'll only need a tiny amount for a great pink punch. If you want more of a pinup red lip gloss just add more carmine, doing little swatch tests as you go until you get a color you like.

MAKES APPROXIMATELY 1.5 OUNCES (43 G) LIP GLOSS

1 recipe Lip Gloss Base, beeswax or vegan, prepared (page 156)

$^{1}/_{16}$ teaspoon carmine

10 to 15 drops essential oils (optional; I'd recommend peppermint)

Bronze Shimmer Lip Gloss

FOR THIS LIP GLOSS WE'LL USE BRONZE MICA TO GET A SHIMMERY, LIGHTLY TINTED SUN-KISSED LIP GLOSS.

MAKES APPROXIMATELY 1.5 OUNCES (43 G) LIP GLOSS

1 recipe Lip Gloss Base, beeswax or vegan, prepared (page 156)

$^{3}/_{16}$ teaspoon bronze mica

10 to 15 drops essential oils (optional; I'd recommend peppermint)

Autumn Lip Gloss

A BLEND OF WARM RED AND YELLOW OXIDES COMBINED WITH SOME GOLD MICA MAKES FOR A LIP GLOSS that's reminiscent of warm fall days and pumpkin spice lattes.

MAKES APPROXIMATELY 1.5 OUNCES (43 G) LIP GLOSS

1 recipe Lip Gloss Base, beeswax or vegan, prepared (page 156)

$1/16$ teaspoon red iron oxide

$3/64$ teaspoon yellow iron oxide

$3/32$ teaspoon gold mica

10 to 15 drops essential oils (optional; I'd recommend peppermint)

INVENT YOUR OWN!

To create your own lip gloss color blends start with about $1/16$ teaspoon of pigment per batch of lip gloss base, but there really aren't any hard or fast rules—just play, have fun, and take notes so you can recreate your favorites!

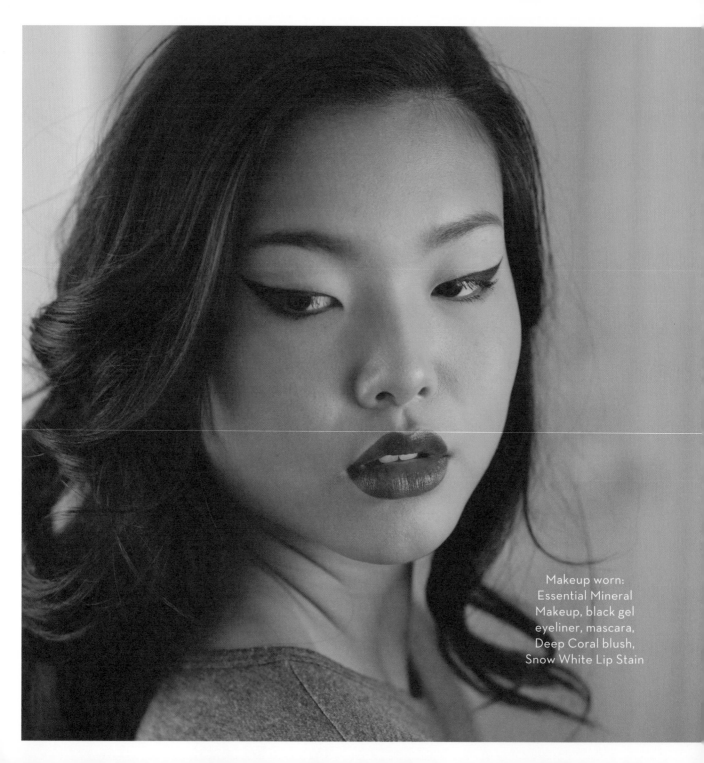

Makeup worn:
Essential Mineral
Makeup, black gel
eyeliner, mascara,
Deep Coral blush,
Snow White Lip Stain

Snow White Lip Stain

WHEN I CALL SOMETHING A LIP STAIN, I'M NOT FOOLING AROUND. THIS CARMINE-POWERED LIP STAIN PACKS a seriously colorful punch and can last all day (it also doubles as a fantastic cheek stain!). Because it's highly pigmented, but still translucent, it looks amazing on all skin tones; it simply adds red to your lip color, rather than replacing your lip color with something new. I think you'll love it.

I spent over a year experimenting with different natural colorants to make a proper lip stain. I was daydreaming about something that would properly stain my lips. A thin, vibrantly pigmented water-based liquid that could be painted on. It would sink into the lips and deliver pure, fantastic color all day long. I'd been disappointed by shop-bought so-called "stains" I'd tried, and I wanted something amazing.

In order for the stain to really stain, the pigment needed to be soluble, so iron oxides and clays were out. I tried a lot of different colorful plant-based powders and extracts in my quest for my dream lip stain—everything from dark red beetroot powder to hot pink rosehip extract. Nothing worked. Every attempt at a stain was roughly as pigmented as a cup of tea—capable of staining a dish towel, but not lips. To add insult to injury, the plant-based pigments would quickly oxidize and the color would shift from red to a sad, murky brown in a matter of days.

And then I discovered carmine. If you could have been a fly on the wall when I first gave it a go, you'd have thought I won the lottery—there was quite a bit of energetic jumping about and squealing. Carmine is amazing. It's incredibly potent, and a fantastic shade of bright pinup red. It's been used as a red pigment for centuries—the Aztecs used it for dying and painting! It's made from the cochineal beetle, so while carmine is natural, it is not vegan. The vibrant, potent color of carmine is unmatched elsewhere in nature, though D&C Red Lake No. 7 is a close synthetic color match. Red Lake No. 7 is though, so it's not a suitable alternative to carmine in lip stain, meaning there is no vegan way to make this lip stain.

My Snow White Lip Stain packs a bright red punch of color that's fantastic for all-day wear. A base of vibrantly pigmented carmine is mixed with water and glycerin to make a richly colored stain that can be painted onto the lips. Glycerin adds a bit of sweetness to the mixture, as well as helping hydrate the lips by attracting moisture to them.

We'll be making lip stain in small amounts, but once you see how potent it is, you'll understand why. Thanks to these small batch sizes you'll need fairly little carmine, so if you happen to find a supplier that sells sample packs of carmine (under 0.17 ounce [5 g]), one of those will be plenty for several batches of lip stain.

   To avoid having your wee bit of lip stain rolling around in a giant container, I'd recommend looking for 0.17 ounce (5 g) plastic jars with sealing lids. They're a great size and pretty cute to boot! I like to make the lip stain in the same container I store it in to cut back on mess.

MAKES APPROXIMATELY
0.07 FLUID OUNCE (2 ML)

$1/16$ teaspoon carmine

12 drops vegetable glycerin

10 drops water

Broad-spectrum preservative (follow manufacturer's recommendation for usage amount; if your preservative is liquid, one drop will be more than enough)

Measure the carmine, vegetable glycerin, water, and preservative out into the small jar you plan on storing the lip stain in, and gently stir everything together with a toothpick until the mixture is smooth and uniform (this will take about 1 minute). That's it! It'll take a bit of convincing to get the carmine to wet out and incorporate, but it will—just keep stirring.

   To use, apply the stain to dry, exfoliated lips with a lip brush. Because this lip stain is entirely water-based it will bead up and run off your lips if you've recently applied lip balm or another oily/waxy product, so your lips should be naked, but not flaky.

   The lip stain is really potent, so start off with pretty small amounts, blending it in and layering up. Once I'm done applying the stain to my lips, I like to dab my cheeks with what remains on the brush and quickly blend that in with my fingertips for a beautiful cheek stain. When the lip stain has dried it's pretty durable, so go ahead and put softer lip balm (like my Naked Lip Balm on page 49) or lip gloss on over top.

   Because this lip stain contains water, it can spoil, which is why we've included a broad-spectrum preservative. If you notice any changes in terms of scent, texture, color, or perhaps the appearance of a fuzzy mold colony, chuck it out and make a fresh batch.

LIPSTICK

Gone are the days where you agonize over which shade of lipstick to buy at the shops—you can have them all, and more! Homemade lipstick is a step up from homemade tinted lip balm in the color department. There's obviously far more pigment to create deep, vibrant colors, so the base recipe is tweaked a bit to include magnesium stearate and magnesium myristate for better adhesion and slip (all those powdery pigments can make for a lipstick that's unpleasantly skiddy). Once you've got your base, the only limit to the colors you can blend is your imagination (and the size of your pigment collection, of course).

Each base recipe makes enough to produce about eight 0.17 ounce (5 g) pots of lipstick (for reference, most shop-bought lipsticks are 0.1 to 0.15 ounce [3 to 4.25 g]). Rather than making eight tubes of identical lipstick, though, I'd really recommend dividing up the base to make a few different colors. Each 0.17 ounce (5 g) of lipstick base requires $7/16$ teaspoon of pigment, so you can blend $7/16$ teaspoon of pigment together and combine it with 0.17 ounce (5 g) of lipstick base in a small dish before melting and blending everything together to make just one pot of lipstick. This is a great way to experiment with different colors. Be sure to take notes on all your different color blends so you can replicate your favorites later!

Blending powdered pigments into the lipstick base is easily the most time-consuming part of making lipstick—it will take at least 3 to 5 minutes of smooshing, stirring, and mashing your lipstick around to get an even color blend (lipstick color blending is much more time-consuming than creamy eyeliner color blending because of the frequent inclusion of clumpy, hard-to-blend titanium dioxide in lipstick colors). If you want to cut back on your pigment blending time, give your pigments a thorough blitz in your coffee grinder. Remember to sandwich a piece of plastic wrap between the grinder and the lid so you don't lose a lot of pigment to the inside of the coffee grinder. After you've ground your pigments together for a solid 20 to 30 seconds, add the blended pigments to 0.17 ounce (5 g) of lipstick base and proceed as usual. Make sure you get as much pigment as possible out of the grinder and into your lipstick base (a small, fluffy cosmetics brush is really helpful) so you don't end up with a noticeably less pigmented final product. This extra step will easily cut your blending time in half and will provide a much better blend than you'll achieve with stirring and smooshing alone. The difference in the final lipstick isn't so noticeable that you should feel like it's necessary, but you'll love this extra step if you're a bit of a perfectionist!

Long-Wear Lipstick Base

THIS FANTASTIC BASE MAKES A LIPSTICK THAT IS IMPERVIOUS TO GLASSWARE, HANDILY STICKING AROUND through several pints or a pot of tea. This formula was actually born out of some earlier experiments in oil-based eyeliner, which led to a rather curious-looking me wandering around my house for a day wearing some eyeliner as a shockingly dark impromptu lipstick.

I've found this lipstick can be applied at the start of the work day and still look pretty good by the time I get home in the evening. Testers said they stopped counting at 9 hours of wear. It's sturdy enough to apply a softer lip balm (like my Naked Lip Balm on page 49) over top of it throughout the day, keeping lips hydrated and happy.

MAKES EIGHT 0.17 OUNCE (5 G) POTS OF LIPSTICK

0.35 ounce (10 g) refined beeswax	10 drops vitamin E oil
0.1 ounce (3 g) candelilla wax	1 teaspoon magnesium stearate
0.46 ounce (13 g) castor oil	³/₄ teaspoon magnesium myristate
0.46 ounce (13 g) jojoba oil	

Creamy Vegan Lipstick Base

FOR A CREAMIER ALTERNATIVE, TRY THIS VEGAN BASE, MADE WITH COCOA BUTTER, COCONUT OIL, AND sweet almond oil. Since it's softer than the long-wear variety it doesn't stay on quite as long, but you should still get 4 to 6 hours of wear without touch-ups.

MAKES EIGHT 0.17 OUNCE (5 G) POTS OF LIPSTICK

0.35 ounce (10 g) candelilla wax	10 drops vitamin E oil
0.25 ounce (7 g) cocoa butter	1³/₄ teaspoon magnesium stearate
0.35 ounce (10 g) coconut oil	1 teaspoon magnesium myristate
0.53 ounce (15 g) sweet almond oil or safflower oil	Pigment (see Lipstick Color Blends section on page 167)

To make either lipstick base, weigh the waxes, butters, oils, magnesium stearate, and magnesium myristate into a small saucepan and stir everything together with a flexible silicone spatula, breaking up the clumps of magnesium stearate and magnesium myristate and thoroughly blending the powders into the oils so everything will melt evenly. Place the saucepan over low heat to melt slowly; this will take about 30 minutes. The reason we aren't using a water bath here is because magnesium stearate melts at 190°F (88°C), and while that is below the temperature of boiling water (212°F [100°C]), I find it's quite difficult to get magnesium stearate to melt in a water bath, while it melts easily over direct heat. Watch your lipstick base carefully as it melts so you don't accidentally scorch it; if you do, you'll want to chuck it and start over as your lipstick will end up looking strangely curdled when you add the pigment as well as smelling and tasting pretty awful.

As the base melts you'll reach a point where it's liquid, but appears cloudy—that's unmelted magnesium stearate and magnesium myristate. The base hasn't fully melted until that cloudiness disappears and you're left with a transparent golden liquid. You'll probably have a bit of foam on top, but that will go away when you remove the base from the heat and start working with it.

Once everything has melted your base is done!

If you want to make it into lipstick right away you can, but you can also pour the base into a small jar and save it for use at a later date (it'll last at least a year if stored somewhere cool and dry).

Now it's time to start adding pigment!
To turn your base into lipstick, start by preparing a hot water bath by heating approximately 1 inch (2.5 cm) of water in a wide, shallow pan. You don't want it to be simmering, just steaming hot—that way the lipstick base will melt, but the bubbling water won't toss the dish around and potentially bounce into your lipstick.

Up next, weigh 0.17 ounce (5 g) of lipstick base into a small bowl (aim for something that holds half a cup [125 mL] or less) and add your pigments. Place that bowl into your hot water bath to melt the base (and keep it melted) so you can blend in the pigment. I find a thin, flexible silicone spatula to be the best tool for pigment blending; you can use it to smear the pigments up against the sides and bottom of the dish to break them up. This will take longer than you'd think—feel free to remove the bowl from the water bath to blend without steaming yourself, popping the bowl of lipstick back into the hot water bath as needed to keep everything melted enough to stir. As you draw your spatula across the bottom of the bowl, you'll be able to see streaks of bright pigments as they break down and blend in, and you'll keep seeing streaks after several minutes of smearing and stirring. Keep at it—after 3 to 5 minutes of blending those streaks will all but disappear (see page 163 for tips on reducing this blending time).

Once you've got a smooth, evenly pigmented lipstick, you're done! If you'd like to blend in a drop or two of an essential oil (peppermint is nice) now's the time, otherwise it's time to pour your lipstick into a 0.17 ounce (5 g) (or larger) pot or a 0.15 ounce (4.25 g) lip balm tube. I prefer pots as I like to apply lipstick with a lip brush, but tubes certainly make for easier on-the-go application.

Let your lipstick solidify before using. It will only take about 10 minutes to solidify enough to use, but it will continue to harden for up to 24 hours after you pour it, so don't be surprised if it seems too soft at first!

Because this lipstick is entirely oil-based, we're not worried about it molding, though the oils can oxidize and go rancid. The vitamin E in the base will help prevent that, so you can expect a shelf life of about a year if your lipstick is stored somewhere relatively cool and dry. If you notice your lip balm starts to smell like crayons or old nuts, that's a sign the oils have oxidized, and it's time to chuck it out and make a fresh one.

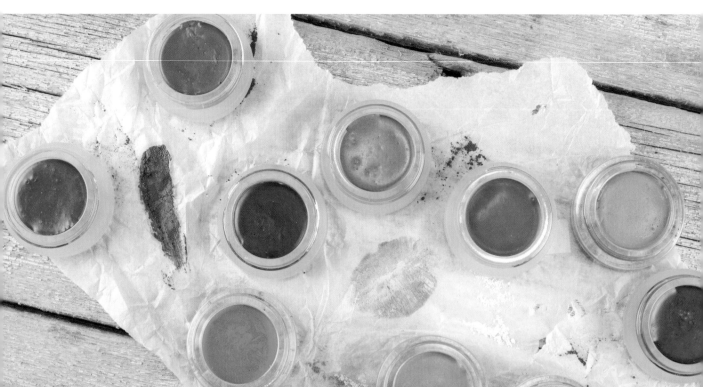

LIPSTICK COLOR BLENDS

Red Dahlia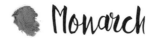

A CLASSIC DEEP RED, REMINISCENT OF OLD HOLLYWOOD AND GLAMOUR.

0.17 ounce (5 g) Lipstick Base, Long-Wear or
Creamy Vegan, prepared (page 164)

$1/4$ teaspoon carmine

$3/32$ teaspoon red iron oxide, blue shade

$3/32$ teaspoon titanium dioxide

Monarch

THIS ALMOST-CORAL IS MOSTLY RED WITH THE
faintest tint of orange and just a hint of golden shimmer.

0.17 ounce (5 g) Lipstick Base, Long-Wear or
Creamy Vegan, prepared (page 164)

$7/32$ teaspoon carmine

$1/16$ teaspoon red iron oxide

$1/16$ teaspoon yellow iron oxide

$1/8$ teaspoon titanium dioxide

$1/8$ teaspoon gold mica

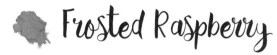

Frosted Raspberry

AN ULTRA-WEARABLE RASPBERRY TONE THAT'S GREAT YEAR-ROUND.

0.17 ounce (5 g) Lipstick Base, Long-Wear
or Creamy Vegan, prepared (page 164)

$^1/_4$ teaspoon titanium dioxide

$^3/_{32}$ teaspoon carmine

$^3/_{32}$ teaspoon red iron oxide

Blushing Taupe

A CLASSIC NUDE FOR LIGHTER COMPLEXIONS WITH A HINT OF WARM BLUSH.

0.17 ounce (5 g) Lipstick Base, Long-Wear
or Creamy Vegan, prepared (page 164)

$^{11}/_{32}$ teaspoon titanium dioxide

$^3/_{64}$ teaspoon red iron oxide

$^3/_{64}$ teaspoon yellow iron oxide

$^1/_8$ teaspoon bronze mica

Nude Coral

A LOVELY LIGHT NUDE WITH A HINT OF CORAL AND SHIMMER.

0.17 ounce (5 g) Lipstick Base, Long-Wear
or Creamy Vegan, prepared (page 164)

$^1/_{16}$ teaspoon carmine

$^1/_8$ teaspoon yellow iron oxide

$^1/_4$ teaspoon titanium dioxide

$^1/_{16}$ teaspoon gold mica

Summer Coral

A BRIGHT CORAL THAT'S PERFECT WITH SUMMER DRESSES AND PATIO COCKTAILS.

0.17 ounce (5 g) Lipstick Base, Long-Wear
or Creamy Vegan, prepared (page 164)

$3/32$ teaspoon carmine

$3/16$ teaspoon yellow iron oxide

$5/32$ teaspoon titanium dioxide

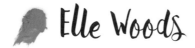

Elle Woods

A CLASSIC BRIGHT PINK LIPSTICK THAT
brings up memories of glitter and scrunchies.

0.17 ounce (5 g) Lipstick Base, Long-Wear
or Creamy Vegan, prepared (page 164)

$1/4$ teaspoon titanium dioxide

$1/8$ teaspoon carmine

$1/16$ teaspoon yellow iron oxide

Blackberry Sorbet

A DEEP, COOL PLUM WITH A HINT OF SILVERY SHIMMER.

0.17 ounce (5 g) Lipstick Base, Long-Wear
or Creamy Vegan, prepared (page 164)

$5/32$ teaspoon carmine

$5/32$ teaspoon blue ultramarine

$1/16$ teaspoon red iron oxide

$1/16$ teaspoon titanium dioxide

$1/8$ teaspoon silver mica

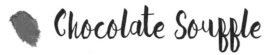

Chocolate Soufflé

A DEEP WARM CHOCOLATE BROWN THAT
makes a beautiful nude on darker skin tones.

0.17 ounce (5 g) Lipstick Base, Long-Wear
or Creamy Vegan, prepared (page 164)

$^1/_{16}$ teaspoon titanium dioxide

$^3/_{16}$ teaspoon brown iron oxide

$^1/_8$ teaspoon red iron oxide

$^1/_{16}$ teaspoon yellow iron oxide

Adore

NAMED FOR AND INSPIRED BY MY FRIEND ADORA,
this stunning deep shade is cool perfection on dark skin tones.

0.17 ounce (5 g) Lipstick Base, Long-Wear
or Creamy Vegan, prepared (page 164)

$^1/_{16}$ teaspoon titanium dioxide

$^3/_{16}$ teaspoon brown iron oxide

$^3/_{16}$ teaspoon blue ultramarine

INVENT YOUR OWN!

Ready to dive into blending your own lipstick colors? The rule of thumb is $^7/_{16}$ teaspoon of pigment per 0.17 ounce (5 g) lipstick base (not including micas), but you can definitely experiment with more or less pigment and see what you think!

LIP PAINT

This fantastic lip paint is incredibly easy to make, highly pigmented, and stays on like a charm. It easily lasts upward of 4 to 6 hours, through drinks, meals, and even brushing your teeth. I wore it to an Irish whiskey tasting and didn't leave a lip print on a single glass! You can easily apply lip balm or lip gloss over top of it to keep lips feeling hydrated through your marathon color session. It's good stuff.

Whenever you remove wax from a lipstick you start to encounter some pretty serious color-bleeding problems. Earlier versions of this lip paint would crawl off my lips and spiderweb down my chin and up toward my nose like a tiny network of red rivers. Perfect for a creepy zombie costume, but less useful for daily wear. A quick and simple addition of calcium carbonate, which is crazy absorbent even in small quantities, helps nail the color to the confines of your lips.

To extend the staying power I added magnesium stearate and magnesium myristate. Both help immensely with adhesion, and magnesium stearate has the added benefit of improving slip as well.

The final product is like a thick oil paint. A little goes a very long way, and can be blended into the lips for more of a stained look or layered up for a full coverage color pop. You might find it's a bit drying; you can remedy that by gently applying lip balm on top after it sets, or by adding another one or two drops of castor oil to the base blend. The more oil you add to the base the softer it will be, meaning that it won't apply as precisely and will be more likely to bleed, but it also won't be as drying.

Note: Ultramarines are not approved for use on the lips in the United States, but they are allowed in the European Union. Given the European Union's approval I have included some ultramarines in a few lip colors, but if you are uncomfortable using it, FD&C Blue No. 1 Aluminum Lake is a good alternative that is approved for use on the lips in both the United States and the European Union.

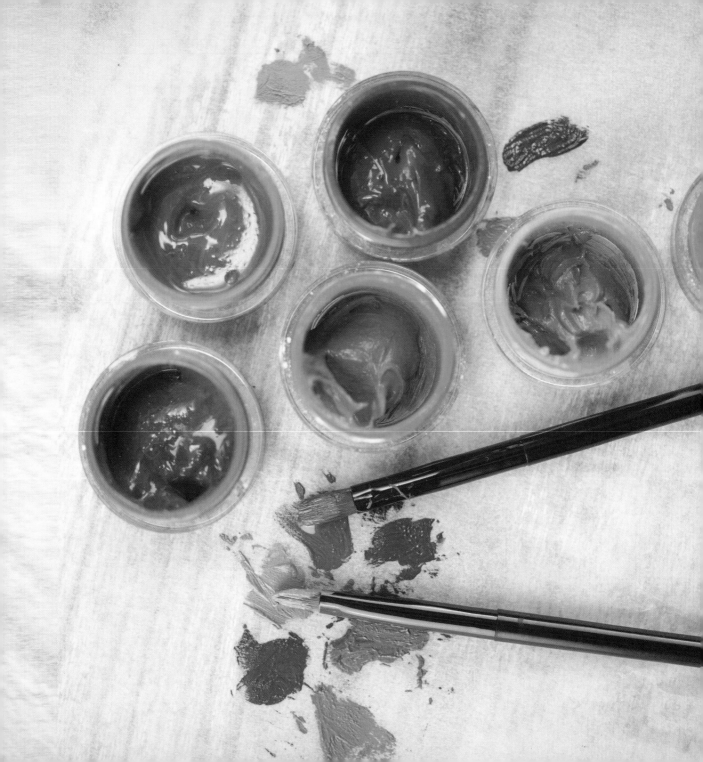

Lip Paint Base

MAKES APPROXIMATELY 0.07
OUNCE (2 G)

$^1/_{16}$ **teaspoon magnesium stearate**

$^1/_{16}$ **teaspoon magnesium myristate**

$^3/_{32}$ **teaspoon calcium carbonate**

16 drops castor oil

12 drops jojoba oil

4 drops vitamin E oil

**Pigment (see Lip Paint Color
  Blends section on page 174)**

Start with a 0.17 ounce (5 g) jar with a sealing lid; we'll mix everything in one and then just leave it in there for as little cleanup as possible.

Measure all the powders out into the jar—magnesium stearate, magnesium myristate, calcium carbonate, and all your pigments from one of my color blends (or your own!). Carefully stir the powders together with a toothpick, and then add the oils. Gently stir everything together, swirling the oils in the center of the pot and allowing them to pull the powders in gradually—if you dive in too enthusiastically you'll spray the powders out of the container and make a mess. After a minute or so of stirring, you'll end up with a thick, highly pigmented paste. That's it!

Because this lip paint is entirely oil-based we aren't worried about mold, though the oils can oxidize and go rancid. Vitamin E is a powerful antioxidant and will help prevent this, so your lip paints should keep for at least a year if stored somewhere relatively cool and dry. If you notice your lip paint starts to smell off, like crayons or old nuts, that's an indication that the oils have oxidized; throw it out and make a fresh batch.

LIP PAINT COLOR BLENDS

Berry Red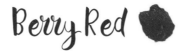

THIS CLASSIC, COOL RED HUE ALSO MAKES A
beautiful cream blush. Pair with a cat eye for best results.

1 recipe Lip Paint Base, unprepared (page 173)

$1/16$ teaspoon titanium dioxide

$1/16$ teaspoon red iron oxide

$1/8$ teaspoon carmine

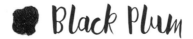 # Black Plum

A VERSATILE, COOL PURPLY TONE THAT SHIFTS COLOR AS YOU
layer it up; use a little for a cool red or work up to a lovely, wearable plum.

1 recipe Lip Paint Base, unprepared (page 173)

$1/16$ teaspoon titanium dioxide

$1/16$ teaspoon red iron oxide, blue shade

$1/8$ teaspoon carmine

Mini Skirt

THIS PERFECT SUMMERY PINK WILL SEND YOU
searching for a cute dress and your favorite flats.

1 recipe Lip Paint Base, unprepared (page 173)

$1/16$ teaspoon carmine

$1/8$ teaspoon yellow iron oxide

$1/16$ teaspoon titanium dioxide

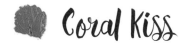

Coral Kiss

PERFECTLY BALANCED BETWEEN CORAL AND NUDE,
this highly wearable shade is downright beautiful.

1 recipe Lip Paint Base, unprepared (page 173)

$1/32$ teaspoon carmine

$1/8$ teaspoon yellow iron oxide

$3/32$ teaspoon titanium dioxide

$1/32$ teaspoon gold mica (optional—adds shimmer)

Tickled Pink

A HOT PINK COLOR POP TO BRIGHTEN ANY DAY.

1 recipe Lip Paint Base, unprepared (page 173)

$1/16$ teaspoon titanium dioxide

$1/16$ teaspoon carmine

$1/16$ teaspoon silver mica (optional—adds shimmer)

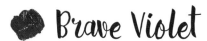 # Brave Violet

THIS COOL, EYE-CATCHING PURPLE IS NOT FOR THE FAINT OF HEART.

1 recipe Lip Paint Base, unprepared (page 173)

$^1/_{16}$ teaspoon carmine

$^3/_{32}$ teaspoon blue ultramarine

$^1/_{16}$ teaspoon titanium dioxide

···· INVENT YOUR OWN! ····

Want to blend up your own lip paint colors? The rule of thumb is $^1/_4$ teaspoon pigment per recipe of Lip Paint Base (page 173), with up to $^1/_{16}$ teaspoon of mica on top of that if you want some shimmer.

Tip: Looking for some brighter colors to work with? Take a look at the D&C Lake pigments; they're available in a variety of reds, blues, yellows, and oranges that are much brighter than iron oxides, and with similar safety ratings on the Environmental Working Group's Skin Deep database (generally 1/10, while oxides score 2/10). Try swapping the yellow iron oxide in a coral lipstick for an equal amount of FD&C Yellow No. 5 or No. 10 for a much brighter final product, or swap carmine out for D&C Red Lake No. 7 for a much cheaper alternative.

STOCKISTS AND SUPPLIERS

UNITED STATES

Bramble Berry
   http://www.brambleberry.com/

Bulk Apothecary
   http://www.bulkapothecary.com/

Bulk Herb Store
   http://www.bulkherbstore.com/

Essential Depot
   http://www.essentialdepot.com/

Essential Wholesale & Labs
   http://www.essentialwholesale.com/

Formulator Sample Shop
   http://www.formulatorsampleshop.com

Ingredients to Die For
   http://www.ingredientstodiefor.com/

Lotion Crafter
   http://www.lotioncrafter.com/

Making Cosmetics
   http://www.makingcosmetics.com/

Mountain Rose Herbs
   https://www.mountainroseherbs.com/

New Directions Aromatics (*recommended*)
   http://newdirectionsaromatics.com/

Nurture Soap
   https://nurturesoap.com/

Soap Goods
   https://www.soapgoods.com

SKS Bottle & Packaging, Inc.
   https://www.sks-bottle.com/

TKB Trading (*recommended*)
   https://www.howtomakecosmetics.com

Wholesale Supplies Plus
   http://www.wholesalesuppliesplus.com/

CANADA

Candora Soap
   http://www.candorasoap.ca/

Canwax
   http://www.canwax.com/

New Directions Aromatics (*recommended*)
   http://www.newdirectionsaromatics.ca

Saffire Blue (*recommended*)
   http://saffireblue.ca/

Voyageur Soap & Candle
   http://www.voyageursoapandcandle.com/

Windy Point Soap Making Supplies
  (*recommended*)
  http://www.windypointsoap.com/
YellowBee
  http://yellowbee.ca/

CANADA (FRENCH)

Coop Coco
  https://coopcoco.ca/
Herbularius
  http://herbularius.com/
Les Âmes Fleurs
  http://www.lesamesfleurs.com/
Saffire Blue (*recommended*)
  http://www.saffireblue.ca/shop/fr/

EUROPE

Aromantic (UK)
  http://www.aromantic.co.uk
Gracefruit (UK)
  http://www.gracefruit.com
Just a Soap (UK)
  http://www.justasoap.co.uk
Mystic Moments (UK)
  http://www.mysticmomentsuk.com/
Naissance (UK)
  http://www.enaissance.co.uk/essential-oils
New Directions Aromatics (UK)
  http://www.newdirectionsuk.com/
The Soap Kitchen (UK)

http://www.thesoapkitchen.co.uk
Aroma-Zone (France)
  http://www.aroma-zone.com
Behawe (Germany)
  http://www.behawe.com
Dragonspice Naturwaren (Germany)
  http://www.dragonspice.de
Kosmetikmacherei (Austria)
  http://www.kosmetikmacherei.at/
Waldehoe (Austria)
  http://www.waldehoe.at/
De Hekserij (The Netherlands)
  http://www.hekserij.nl
De Online Zeepwinkel (The Netherlands)
  http://www.online-zeepwinkel.nl
Cremas Caseras (Spain)
  http://www.cremas-caseras.es/

AUSTRALIA AND NEW ZEALAND

Heirloom Body Care (Australia)
  http://www.heirloombodycare.com.au
N Essentials (Australia)
  http://www.n-essentials.com.au/
New Directions Aromatics (Australia)
  http://newdirections.com.au/
Southern Skies Soap Supplies (Australia)
  http://southernskiessoapsupplies.com.au
Go Native (New Zealand)
  http://www.gonative.co.nz

FURTHER READING

The Environmental Working Group's Skin Deep Cosmetics Database
  http://www.ewg.org/skindeep
No More Dirty Looks
  http://nomoredirtylooks.com/
Point of Interest!
  http://swiftcraftymonkey.blogspot.ca/
DIY Beauty on Reddit
  https://www.reddit.com/r/DIYBeauty
LisaLise
  http://www.lisaliseblog.com/

MAKEUP APPLICATION

Lisa Eldridge
  http://www.lisaeldridge.com/
  https://www.youtube.com/user/lisaeldridgedotcom
Lauren Luke
  https://www.youtube.com/user/panacea81
Pixiwoo Makeup Channel
  https://www.youtube.com/user/pixiwoo
Wayne Goss
  https://www.youtube.com/user/gossmakeupartist

THANKS AND ACKNOWLEDGMENTS

First and foremost I want to thank my readers—all the wonderful people who have supported me at Humblebee & Me over the years. I have learned so much from you, and you always encourage me to learn more and develop the best recipes possible. Your support means the world to me, and is a huge part of why I love making things and sharing my discoveries.

Thank you to my friend Meredith for starting me on the path of natural skin care and cosmetics, and to so many wonderful friends (Sarah, Kara, Jess, Chantal, Harriet, and Craig, to name a few!) for encouraging me as I learn and experiment. I'm endlessly appreciative to the women I worked with to develop color blends and test the cosmetics for this book—Adora, Simone, Monday, Jess, Avneet, and Courtney. Thanks for lending me your faces, your thoughts, and your ideas; they are hugely appreciated. Adrian is owed some serious thanks for checking over the chemistry to make sure I'm not spreading misinformation. I also have to thank my parents and family for their support and encouragement, and for tolerating some pretty absurd messes whenever they visit.

This book wouldn't have happened without my wonderful agent, Kate, who was one of the first people to really see the potential of a cosmetics cookbook. I'm also forever indebted to my amazing editor, Cindy, who enthusiastically embraced my slightly crazy idea (along with the rest of the folks at Running Press) and gave me the chance to make it happen. Thank you to Amanda, my talented book designer, for turning *Make It Up* into a beautiful reality, and to Michael for the wonderful photos from our shoot in Philadelphia.

I couldn't have done this without any of you, and I'm endlessly thankful for your support, insights, encouragements, criticisms, and willingness to let me put things on your faces. You are all wonderful.

INDEX

Page numbers in italics refer to photographs.

Notes